"I found *Yoga on Prescription* bo
Fox generously share the scienti
Yoga4Health series and provid
comprehensive course. They offe
efficacy. In addition, they provide collegial support to those of us who don't
live in countries that currently social prescribe. I especially appreciated their
encouragement for us as yoga teachers and therapists to draw upon their model
and feel empowered to integrate therapeutic yoga into the mainstream medical
system by creating similar programming within our own communities."

— *Robin Rothenberg, yoga therapist, author of* Restoring
Prana *and Chair of the Accreditation Committee for the
International Association of Yoga Therapists (IAYT)*

"In *Yoga on Prescription*, Paul Fox and Heather Mason provide a timely response
to the mental and physical health consequences of the Covid-19 pandemic. In
their readable book they outline a succinct yoga intervention programme that
may profoundly benefit those whose health has been disrupted by the pandemic.
The book provides the public health justification for their intervention, which
can be efficiently implemented on the chair or the mat, as well as a plausible
explanation of how yoga would enhance health."

— *Dr Stephen Porges, Professor of Psychiatry at the University of
North Carolina and author of* The Polyvagal Theory

"Restoring health and successfully managing lifestyle-related disorders is
presented in *Yoga on Prescription (The Yoga4Health Social Prescribing Protocol)*
by Paul Fox and Heather Mason, which makes for an informative and interesting
read. This book combines traditional principles of yoga with research-based
guidelines for practice and addresses a much-felt need in integrative healthcare."

— *Shirley Telles, Director, Patanjali Research Foundation, Haridwar, India*

"Yoga for better health – like the approach presented in this book – has the
potential to transform the lives of millions of people through embracing
functional breathing from three dimensions; biochemical, biomechanical and
cadence breathing. Having a deeper understanding can impart the wisdom to
open airways, improve blood circulation, increase oxygen delivery and balance
the nervous system."

— *Patrick McKeown, Clinical Director, Buteyko Clinic
International, author of* The Breathing Cure

"Worldwide healthcare is undergoing a paradigm shift driven partially by necessity stemming from the prevailing broken system but also by innovative pioneers who clearly see the virtue of fostering health instead of treating disease. They can help us envision a path forward that optimally combines both modern invention and time-tested approaches heretofore bypassed by mainstream medicine.

Yoga on Prescription by Paul Fox and Heather Mason is an important contribution to this process. It not only provides compelling empirical evidence but also a lucid explanation of how therapeutic yoga fits and functions within the realm of social prescribing and patient activation. For those interested in the real-world aspects of the health paradigm shift, this is a must read."

– James Marzolf, Senior Director, Health Sector
Finance & Policy, Whole Health Institute

"This gem of a book, which very well could prove to be one of the most important books of this decade, gives us the essence of yoga as a possible modern-day prescription for real health. As Sat Bir Khalsa puts it in the foreword, our modern acute care healthcare system model is so focused on symptom treatment, dominated by technological approaches including pharmaceuticals and surgery. Heather Mason and Paul Fox have done an amazing job – this book is a clear glass of water, refreshing in its simplicity!"

– Goran Boll, creator of MediYoga in the Swedish public healthcare system

"Bringing yoga into social prescription is a stroke of genius. Occupying the ground between specialized medicine and general wellbeing, it tackles the biggest problem facing modern healthcare – unhealthy lifestyles. The UK is ideally situated to pioneer this approach because its National Health Service reaches everyone – and within reach of nearly everyone there are yoga teachers who are competent to hold suitable yoga classes, given a little specialized training for which this is the course book."

– Dr Robin Monro, founder of the UK yoga therapy profession

"This book provides an excellent overview of the history of yoga practices and applications to health, as well as the recent scientific advances explaining modern understanding of the underlying mechanisms, by which yoga can improve physical and mental health. This book can be used as a useful tool for teaching to appreciate the therapeutic benefits of yoga and training of healthcare practitioners and students who want to integrate yoga therapy into their clinical practices."

– Dr Helen Lavretsky, Professor of Psychiatry, UCLA

"Yoga4Health, through Paul and Heather's innovation and passion, is at the forefront of bringing yoga and its wide range of benefits, safely into our healthcare systems on prescription. This evidence-based protocol targets not only prevention, but also treatment of chronic disease, while working in conjunction with modern medicine."

– Dr Avi Sharma, GP, Kilmarnock

"This detailed (but at the same time eminently readable) book is a trailblazer that describes the rapidly developing acceptance of the use of appropriate yoga in the management of common lifestyle conditions. Undoubtedly, this ground-breaking work will be a reference source, an inspiration and a guide for all advocates and practitioners of lifestyle medicine."

– Dr Ruth Gilmore, yoga therapist, anatomy teacher, and author of Ask Ruth

"This methodical book serves as a great resource for people working in the health and wellness sectors in a number of ways. It not only provides a literature overview of the growing base of research to support the profound restorative power of yoga; it also illustrates the importance of not reducing yoga to a mere physical practice. As the NHS takes on its greatest transformation in decades, this book demonstrates the tremendous potential of social prescribing. Including yoga in social prescribing will make the practice more accessible to underserved communities and support their ability to take control of their own health and wellbeing. This serves as one essential step in reducing health inequities in society."

– Dr Stacie CC Graham, author of Yoga as
Resistance *and founder of OYA Retreats*

YOGA ON PRESCRIPTION

The Yoga4Health Social Prescribing Protocol

PAUL FOX and HEATHER MASON

Foreword by Sat Bir Singh Khalsa

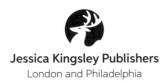

Jessica Kingsley Publishers
London and Philadelphia

First published in Great Britain in 2022 by Jessica Kingsley Publishers
An imprint of Hodder & Stoughton Ltd
An Hachette Company

1

Disclaimer: *The information contained in this book is not intended to replace the services of
trained medical professionals or to be a substitute for medical advice. The complementary therapy
described in this book may not be suitable for everyone to follow. You are advised to consult a
doctor before embarking on any complementary therapy programme and on any matters relating
to your health, and in particular on any matters that may require diagnosis or medical attention.*

A CIP catalogue record for this title is available from the
British Library and the Library of Congress

ISBN 978 1 78775 975 6
eISBN 978 1 78775 976 3

Printed and bound in Great Britain by TJ Books Limited

Jessica Kingsley Publishers' policy is to use papers that are natural, renewable
and recyclable products and made from wood grown in sustainable
forests. The logging and manufacturing processes are expected to conform
to the environmental regulations of the country of origin.

Jessica Kingsley Publishers
Carmelite House
50 Victoria Embankment
London EC4Y 0DZ

www.jkp.com

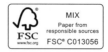

Contents

Foreword

Yoga researcher Sat Bir Singh Khalsa, PhD, Assistant Professor of Medicine, Harvard Medical School

Unequivocally, the biggest burden in healthcare in terms of its negative impact on mortality, healthcare costs, medical and psychological symptoms, longevity, wellness and quality of life is the worldwide epidemic of chronic lifestyle-related non-communicable diseases (NCDs). These include cardiovascular diseases, obesity, Type 2 diabetes and even cancer, which is known to be 50% preventable. These disorders are due to the well-known and widespread risk factors of sedentary behaviour, poor dietary habits and unhealthy behaviours, which are exacerbated by an ongoing epidemic of unmanaged chronic stress in modern society. Unfortunately, our modern acute-care healthcare system model is focused primarily on symptom treatment, which is dominated by technological approaches including pharmaceuticals and surgery. There is little focus on a patient-centred, holistic, preventive, integrative and self-care approach to maintaining wellness and addressing the underlying causes of NCDs. It is therefore actually a disease-care system rather than a true healthcare system. Because it does not focus on the risk factors for, and underlying causes of, NCDs, it cannot succeed in effectively addressing the NCD epidemic.

Because NCDs are due to dysfunctional lifestyle behaviours, behaviour change is necessary to prevent and reverse NCDs effectively. Unfortunately, this is not a strength of modern medicine. Often, patients are provided with a list of behaviours they need to change with the motivation of the fear of worsening disease or even premature death;

this is a top-down strategy of attempting to impose behaviour change, and it is not very successful.

As is so thoroughly described in this book, the practice of yoga provides workable solutions for the prevention and treatment of NCDs in multiple ways. Through its multicomponent practices of physical postures and exercises, breath-regulation techniques, relaxation practices, and meditation and mindfulness, yoga impacts many physical and psychological characteristics. Significant research has demonstrated its ability to improve stress and emotion regulation, a major contributor to dysfunctional behaviours and NCD risk factors. Over time, with regular practice, the meditative and mindfulness component of yoga improves mind-body awareness or mindfulness, which recent research is showing to be an excellent strategy for behaviour change. By becoming more aware and sensitive to the consequences of their behaviours, patients will start to change behaviour because they wish to avoid the negative sensations and consequences of poor lifestyle behaviours such as sedentary behaviour and junk food. On the other hand, they will be attracted to the positive sensations and rewards of positive health behaviours such as exercise and healthful foods. This is a strategy of behaviour change from the bottom up, and it is becoming well-known that it is more effective. Yoga therefore inherently has a potential for prevention and treatment of NCDs that modern medicine is lacking.

Unfortunately, many modern medical systems, especially multi-payer systems, are not driven by prevention or treatment of underlying causes. As a consequence, in the US, healthcare costs are escalating dramatically, while longevity of the US population is actually falling behind that of other countries. Fortunately, there are examples of medical systems, especially single-payer systems, that are driven to save costs through prevention and behaviour change. These are serving as examples of more holistic and preventive care systems. They include the Veterans Administration medical system in the US, which has incorporated many complementary and integrative medical practices for its patient population, and the NHS in the UK, which has developed the social-prescribing system, which allows for greater patient access to more complementary and integrative practices.

As described fully in this text, the Yoga4Health programme is an excellent model that fits within the NHS social-prescribing system.

The preliminary research of this programme in the UK presented in this book is a very encouraging testament to the efficacy of the Yoga4Health programme in affecting key behaviours relevant to NCDs. We can look forward to the continued successful application and integration of yoga as a valuable practice within the healthcare system. Looking further into the future, the full implementation of yoga practices as a regular and widely accepted mind-body hygiene system within mainstream society, including its regular practice in public schools and workplaces, has great potential for improving prevention of disease and maintenance of overall health and wellbeing.

Acknowledgements

Writing a book is never easy, and this one was no exception. We busted a few deadlines with our snail-like progress! However, we got there in the end, thanks to our family and loved ones. Paul wishes to thank Laura, and his daughters, Jessie, Rosanna and Stephanie, and grandchildren Ada and Leo, for keeping him grounded and sane. Heather would like to thank her family and wonderful teachers along the way.

We both thank our dogs, Minnie Monkey, Mr Whippy and Poppy, for the excuse to take a break from work and tickle-up our vagus nerve with strokes and cuddles.

Professionally, we are indebted to our fellow directors at the Yoga in Healthcare Alliance for their unwavering support: Sat Bir Singh Khalsa, Robin Monro, Nicole Schnackenberg and Sakthi Karunanithi, Dr Avi Sharma, Dr Rupal Dave and Dr Rebekah Lawrence. We also thank Kalwant Sahota and Dr Fiona Butler for having the vision and faith in us to commission the Yoga4Health programme in the first place, and Dr Tina Cartwright and Anna Cheshire for researching our programme and highlighting where things were working or could be improved. Marie Polley also provided sage advice on how to keep the programme in line with social-prescribing guidance.

We are grateful to Tori Williams for design and marketing advice and for masterfully conducting the photoshoot for the Yoga4Health sequence shown in the book, and to Anna Francis for agreeing to be photographed in the postures. Both are talented Yoga4Health teachers and strong forces for good in all that they do.

We thank the team at our publisher, especially Sarah Hamlin for her patience and support.

Those who have worked with Heather and Paul will know how well we complement each other. Throughout this collaboration we have managed to maintain our deep appreciation, respect and love for each other. Long may that continue.

How Yoga Can Transform Health

Health is the greatest gift.

The Buddha

Our state of health is linked closely to the choices we make. Research shows that people who make positive diet and lifestyle changes need less medication and fewer hospital visits (Ornish, 2019). According to Dr Dean Ornish – one of more than 50 progenitors of lifestyle medicine – these positive changes can add up to 14 years of additional life.

The Yoga4Health protocol presented in this book is designed to help patients put yoga at the centre of a personal lifestyle revolution. Many people need modern medicine when they get sick or a potentially life-saving operation when acute medical problems arise. Alongside the indispensable care that conventional medicine offers, there is a deep (often untapped) potential for patients to help themselves. This self-efficacy, which is intricately tied to self-reliance and personal discipline, leads to patient empowerment. Our aim is to inspire people to adopt a daily yoga practice, to promote greater health and, at the same time, to support positive health behaviours. *Yoga on Prescription* presents a dose of lifestyle medicine that can support health and wellness every day.

As we will see, an increasing body of research reveals that a regular yoga practice can improve physical and mental health, while helping people feel more connected to themselves and those around them. Often, a yogic lifestyle aligns with diet and other changes that support people on their journey to a new and healthier way of living.

Becoming anchored in a daily yoga practice not only nourishes and nurtures the individual; it also has the potential to help society by reducing some of the pressures on overstretched healthcare systems as people more readily take important aspects of their health into their own hands.

Following this introduction, we present the theory and background to the Yoga4Health Yoga on Prescription programme and provide detailed instruction on breathing and a posture-by-posture guide to practising the protocol inclusively on a yoga mat or in a chair.

THE CHALLENGE

Since the advent of antibiotics and other breakthrough biomedical interventions in the first half of the 20th century, the major cause of mortality in the UK has shifted from infectious diseases to lifestyle-related conditions, known as non-communicable diseases (NCDs). It is a similar picture in much of the rest of the world. Sometimes referred to as long-term conditions, NCDs range from various types of heart disease to depressive disorders, cancer, anxiety disorders, lower back pain conditions, Type 2 diabetes, chronic pain conditions, neurodegenerative disorders, chronic obstructive pulmonary disease (COPD), asthma, various autoimmune conditions and others.

The Covid-19 pandemic has served as a reminder that infectious disease can still pose a major threat to human health. However, it was clear early in the pandemic that NCDs still further influenced health, as those with underlying long-term conditions and/or obesity were more likely to be hospitalized and/or die from Covid-19.

According to the World Health Organization (WHO), NCDs contributed to more than 73% of global deaths in 2017 and were a cause of disability across the globe (Ritchie and Roser, 2018). In the same year, cardiovascular disease (including heart attack and stroke) accounted for 18 million deaths (*ibid.*). Nearly 4 million passed away due to respiratory diseases, including COPD and asthma (*ibid.*). Additionally, one third of cancers are linked to lifestyle factors; for example, smoking is the biggest risk factor for lung cancer (Roser and Ritchie, 2021).

Obesity, poor diet, stress, smoking and lack of movement and exercise (or what we will refer to as sedentariness) all increase the risk of developing cardiovascular disease and Type 2 diabetes. WHO data reveals that obesity in men more than trebled between 1975 and 2019 (up from 3.2% to 10.8%), and more than doubled among women (up from 6.4% to 14.9%) (WHO, 2021). WHO also estimates that, in 2019, nearly 2 billion adults were overweight, with 650 million of these clinically obese (*ibid.*). These figures add up to 13% of the world's population.

However, it should be remembered that people can carry more weight and have a range of body shapes and still be healthy.

There is also an obesity crisis in children, with 40 million youngsters under the age of five overweight or obese in 2018 worldwide (*ibid.*). Another 340 million children and adolescents aged 5–19 fall into this category (*ibid.*). In the UK, Public Health England estimates that 29% of adults and 20% of children aged 10–11 are obese (Public Health England, 2021). NHS figures show that, in 2019/20, obesity was linked to more than 11,000 UK hospital admissions and was a factor in a further 876,000 admissions (NHS Digital, 2019).

Those who smoke also face elevated risks of ill health. In the US, up to 90% of all lung cancers are linked to cigarette smoking (Centers for Disease Control and Prevention, 2021a). According to the Centers for Disease Control and Prevention (2021b), smoking cigarettes or exposure to tobacco smoke causes more than 480,000 Americans to die each year from cancer, lung disease, heart disease and stroke.

Apart from the personal and family tragedy associated with premature mortality, NCDs place an enormous burden on healthcare systems. The United Nations (UN) has recognized the importance of this issue, warning that if nothing is done to tackle NCDs, they will cost the global economy 47 trillion dollars by 2030 and the management of them will become untenable for many nations (Duff-Brown, 2017). In September 2015, the UN included the reduction of NCDs in *The 2030 Agenda: For People, Planet and Prosperity*, expounding that NCDs are a sustainable development priority for all countries (NCD Alliance, 2021).

According to The King's Fund, a UK research charity, some 15 million people have a long-term health condition (LTC) (The King's Fund, 2021). The King's Fund estimates that £7 in every £10 of total health and social care spending goes on those with LTCs: "People with long-term conditions now account for about 50% of all GP appointments, 64% of all outpatient appointments and over 70% of all inpatient bed days" (*ibid.*). These patients have earned the moniker "frequent flyers" because they account for so many GP and hospital appointments. Sadly, segments of the population are more prone to LTCs than others, and this requires consideration when drafting health agendas connected to yoga in order to address health inequalities. Age and economic inequality play a big part: 58% of those over the age of 60 present with an LTC, many with more than one; there is a 60% disparity between the highest and lowest socioeconomic groups in those presenting with an LTC (*ibid.*).

Yoga on Prescription is a prevention programme that aspires to support individual journeys towards better health, and in turn reduce the burden on the NHS and health services. The programme is born from a wish both to transform health services and to reduce the health inequities that are correlated with economic inequality by reaching into diverse and marginalized communities. Once we have reached past barriers of access, the solution is often individual; it comes down to the choices people make every day.

A BRIEF HISTORY OF LIFESTYLE MEDICINE

In the 1970s, Dr Dean Ornish began crafting his approach to "Lifestyle Medicine", demonstrating that patients could arrest and even reverse their heart disease through lifestyle changes. In 1993, following extensive research, his Program for Reversing Heart Disease became the first non-surgical and non-pharmaceutical therapy for heart disease to qualify for health-insurance reimbursement in the US.

Dr Ornish's approach has been further bolstered by data from the European Prospective Investigation into Cancer and Nutrition (EPIC), which is following more than half a million participants from ten European countries over 15 years (IARC, 2021).

Research has found that:

Those with four healthy lifestyle factors – moderate exercise of at least 30 minutes per day; not smoking; normal weight; and a high intake of fruits, vegetable, and whole grains and lower meat consumption – reduced the risk of developing any chronic disease by 78%, including a 93% reduction in the risk of Type 2 diabetes, an 81% reduced risk of a heart attack, a 50% reduction in risk for stroke, and a 36% lower risk of developing all forms of cancer. (Ornish, 2019, p.19)

According to Dr Ornish, people following these lifestyle changes lived 12–14 years longer (*ibid.*).

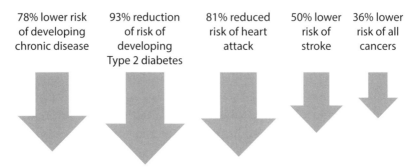

| 78% lower risk of developing chronic disease | 93% reduction of risk of developing Type 2 diabetes | 81% reduced risk of heart attack | 50% lower risk of stroke | 36% lower risk of all cancers |

12–14 years of increased life expectancy – Dr Dean Ornish (2019, p.19)

One of the fundamental points espoused by Dr Ornish is that regardless of the chronic disease a person may have, lifestyle change can help because NCDs share many underlying biological causes, mechanisms and pathways. Lifestyle change can positively affect:

- chronic inflammation and immune system dysfunction

- chronic emotional stress

- gene expression – downregulating (reducing the expression of) genes that cause ill health and upregulating (increasing the expression of) those that enhance health

- telomeres – the ends of DNA strands; greater telomere length is associated with longevity and health

- the microbiome of bacteria in the gut and elsewhere

- cellular resiliency, by reducing oxidative stress.

Dr Ornish has issued a rallying call to fellow doctors urging them to withdraw from "sickcare" in favour of a new paradigm of "healthcare", addressing the underlying causes of ill health. Why keep mopping up the floor, he argues, when it is clear that the cause of the flood is that someone has left on the tap. Turn it off! As the old adage goes, an ounce of prevention is worth a pound of cure. Prevention and early intervention are at the heart of the Yoga4Health programme.

YOGA AND LIFESTYLE CHANGE

Yoga is a comprehensive and integrated system that influences biological, psychological and social aspects of a person to bring about personal transformation. Such interventions are deemed biopsychosocial and are now recognized by modern medicine as crucial in improving health for those with NCDs and to maintain wellbeing in those who are presently healthy but may be at risk due to lifestyle factors. A regular yoga practice (ideally daily) offers a person-centred self-care regime that intelligently and effectively supports people to reach their optimum level of health and wellbeing.

Let's reflect on the incredible growth in popularity of yoga and then consider the scientific evidence illustrating why yoga is such an effective tool for health.

THE YOGA BOOM

Sat Bir Singh Khalsa is Assistant Professor of Medicine at Harvard Medical School and a world-leading yoga researcher (see the foreword to this book). He describes yoga in the US as "a major movement in society" (Khalsa, 2020). The most recent figures show that, in 2017, some 14% of US adults were practising yoga – over 36 million people – and the numbers have continued to increase (The Good Body, 2020).

Worldwide, an estimated 300 million people practise yoga, with around 80% of all practitioners being female (Zuckerman, 2020).

Across the globe, ever-growing numbers of people are attending classes; yoga studios are established in most major towns and cities. Market analysts estimate that the yoga industry was worth 80 billion dollars per annum globally in 2015, and it was projected to grow rapidly during the period to 2026 (Wellness Creative Co, 2021).

But what do we mean by yoga? Many yoga classes include:

- physical postures (*asanas*) used as intelligent exercise

- breathing practices (including traditional yoga breathing techniques known as *pranayama*)

- deep relaxation

- meditation

- yoga philosophy and ideas based on the *yamas* and *niyamas* (behaviours, observances and ways of reappraising thought)

- reflection, awareness and mindfulness.

If we delve into the history of yoga, we find that the path of classical yoga is set out in Patanjali's 2000-year-old text. The *Yoga Sutras of Patanjali* provide a guide for meditating and stilling the mind. This traditional text proclaims that all suffering arises from ignorance within the mind and warped perception.

In the *Yoga Sutras* (which are short verses with deep meaning), Patanjali describes the nature of the mind and the obstacles to settling it so that the true "Self" is revealed. He then sets out a systematic approach to practice, including the eight limbs of yoga known as Ashtanga Yoga (not to be confused with the more recent physical practice of Ashtanga Vinyasa Yoga):

- *yama* – duty, restraint, outer observances

- *niyama* – personal observances, ways of living

- *asana* – posture

- *pranayama* – breathing techniques

- *pratyahara* – sense withdrawal

- *dharana* – concentration

- *dhyana* – meditation

- *samadhi* – a superconscious state of oneness.

This path of Raja (Royal) Yoga was considered a great challenge, requiring dedicated practice and the guidance of a Guru.

By the 15th century, influenced by the Tantra movement, practitioners had developed yoga practices that focused more on the body and breath to prepare for meditation (Muktibodhnananda, 1998). This intermediate step was the birth of Hatha Yoga – the yoga of postures and breathing practices – which accounts for most classes taught today in the Western world.

For centuries, Hatha Yoga and Raja Yoga were practised mainly in

Ashrams in India and among different groups of people there, such as the Naths.

If we fast forward to a house on Versova Beach in Mumbai on Christmas Day 1918, we find the first expression of the modern yoga class (Goldberg, 2016). Shri Yogendra had abandoned his Ashram with the mission to offer yoga techniques to middle-class Indians and their families consisting of postures, breathing techniques and relaxation methods aimed at promoting good health and stress relief. This shift in focus moved yoga from a dedicated spiritual practice to one adapted specifically for health and healing at the level of everyday life. Rather than teach a path to enlightenment, Shri Yogendra wanted to strip yoga of its "mysticism and inertia" (Goldberg, 2016). His formula was exported to the West and steadily took root as more teachers from the East went West, before exploding into popularity over the past 20 years. Following the emerging zeitgeist, in the 1920s Swami Kuvalayananda put yoga under scientific investigation to determine its effects on health, such as the heart rate. He invited Western scientists from prestigious institutions to place yoga under the metaphorical microscope, appreciating that such evidence would both support the transmission of yoga worldwide and offer insight regarding the prescription of specific yoga practices to particular health conditions. Such innovations set the groundwork for others to view yoga as a health system accessible to all.

For a detailed explanation of the historical origins of Hatha Yoga, see *The Path of Modern Yoga* by Elliott Goldberg (2016), *The Yoga Tradition* by Georg Feuerstein (2001) and *Roots of Yoga* by James Mallinson and Mark Singleton (2017). Dr Elizabeth De Michelis, Dr Jason Birch and many academics in India based at universities and organizations like the International Association of Yoga (IAY) continue to build knowledge. Swami Kuvalayananda's organization, Kaivalyadhama (Where Yoga Tradition and Science Meet), continues to flourish.

For a user-friendly approach aimed at the general public, see the Harvard special report, *Introduction to Yoga* (Harvard Medical School, 2021). This publication is a practical introduction for the general public that includes a review of the science and research, as well as recommendations for beginning a yoga practice.

Today, yoga classes cover a broad spectrum, ranging from those that follow a classical comprehensive collection of all the limbs, to classes that focus primarily on movement. These might be physically intense with long holds, flowing movements, gentle postures with controlled breathing or systems devoted only to seated meditation and spiritual self-enquiry. If we are to address the needs of those at risk of becoming chronically ill – and help our health services – gentle forms of healing yoga are usually best suited.

There is also a subfield in yoga, yoga therapy, that uses yoga in managing health complaints. A diploma in yoga therapy could be likened to a Master's degree in yoga for those who want to create tailored programmes for individuals with health conditions. We would argue that there is a form of yoga to suit everyone. The Yoga4Health programme is not yoga therapy, a discipline requiring many additional years of training, but it does straddle the worlds of Hatha Yoga and the therapeutic application of yoga.

Moreover, yoga professionals who are interested in working within systems of healthcare must consider the language that exists therein and the forms of evidence that health systems require. This doesn't mean that yoga loses its roots, but instead (as it has always done) allows itself to be moulded to suit the needs of those who intend to practise it. Yoga has grown spectacularly, but it cannot become embedded in health, education, prisons and the private sector unless it embraces the twin disciplines of high professional standards and evidence-based practice. The world of yoga therapy recognizes how crucial this is and has spent many years developing standards and scope of practice guidelines. The world of yoga professionals wishing to work in healthcare should follow suit, curating relevant guidance and requirements for an intermediate place between the professions of yoga teaching and yoga therapy.

Individuals aspiring to bring yoga into healthcare need comprehensive training relevant to the group they wish to work with and must be familiar with biomedical vernacular, not merely yogic language. In this way, pioneering yoga professionals can translate the benefits of yoga into the very systems they wish to work within. When the Yoga in Healthcare Alliance (YIHA) trains already well-established yoga professionals to bring yoga into healthcare, we highlight important research and discuss the influence of yoga on mental health, the nervous system, the cardiovascular and respiratory systems, anatomical structures and disease. This does not mean that focusing on yoga's energetic effects is not extremely important. It simply means that in healthcare we need to, for the most part, speak in psychophysiological terms and present the evidence base. It also means that we need to let go of unsubstantiated claims about yoga's efficacy, stick with what is scientifically accurate and check our knowledge before parroting something that was told to us about yoga's physiological effects without grounding in research.

In *The Principles and Practice of Yoga in Health Care*, Sat Bir Singh Khalsa is joined by Dr Timothy McCall (author of *Yoga as Medicine*), Lorenzo Cohen and Shirley Telles to summarize over 300 randomized control trials into yoga (Khalsa *et al.*, 2016). The book is a standard text for yoga therapists, and YIHA recommends it to anyone who wants to know more about bringing yoga into healthcare.

Khalsa emphasizes the holistic whole-body and mind effects of yoga: "The yoga practices that we are doing affect us at the cellular and molecular level" (Khalsa, 2020). He also hails the emerging field of psychoneuro-immunology, which examines the effect of the mind on health and resistance to disease, and in particular the interactions between the central nervous system and immune system. Researchers in this area are beginning to link the inability to cope with emotion and stress to impaired immune function.

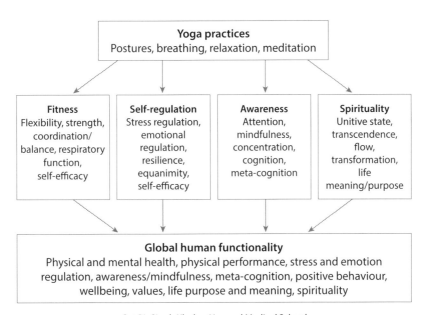

Sat Bir Singh Khalsa, Harvard Medical School

Sat Bir's overview of all the yoga research completed so far (and more studies are being conducted all the time) has led him to reach the conclusion that yoga results in overall improvements in how humans function.

It was the rich and growing evidence base for the positive contribution that yoga can make to health, coupled with a desire to empower people to improve their health, that inspired the creation of YIHA. This UK-based charity has national and global goals to promote yoga's inclusion in health systems. YIHA was established by Heather Mason in 2016 to provide a focal point for the voice of yoga to engage with politicians, policy makers and healthcare professionals. The organization has grown into a nexus for those interested in bringing yoga into healthcare in the UK and beyond.

Alongside YIHA, Heather also established with UK parliamentarians the All-Party Parliamentary Group on Yoga in Society – dedicated to bringing the benefits of yoga into the four pillars of healthcare, schools, prisons and the private sector. Meetings have been held in Parliament with exceptional speakers to brief MPs and peers on the evidence-based benefits of yoga and how yoga can support improvements in society.

YIHA also works closely with the College of Medicine and Integrated Health, whose mission is to promote an integrated approach to healthcare. The College is led by Dr Michael Dixon – a UK pioneer in the field of social prescribing and integrative medicine. He speaks passionately about how doctors need to become responsible for wellness in the communities they serve, not just treating disease. Dr Dixon believes that stepping away from an over-medicalized model means tapping into non-biomedical assets in local communities.

Yoga literally translates as joining/yoking/connecting. It is about bringing things together: body and mind; self and universe; individuals to other individuals, forging wise and healthy communities. Through the Yoga4Health programme, YIHA is working to tap into these non-biomedical assets while working within a biomedical system.

We know yoga works; we know there is a desperate need for the health benefits of yoga to tackle lifestyle-related diseases and reduce pressures on healthcare systems. The mission is to find the best pathway so that healthcare professionals and yoga teachers can work together. Yoga as a social-prescribing intervention has the potential to make a game-changing impact on healthcare, as long as it is backed up by evidence.

A SELECTION OF RESEARCH EVIDENCE

As part of the evaluation of the YIHA Yoga4Health social-prescribing programme, the University of Westminster conducted a review of current available research into the efficacy of yoga, as follows:

Yoga for Cardiovascular Disease and Type 2 Diabetes

Systematic reviews of yoga interventions for patients with cardiovascular disease and Type 2 diabetes show a range of significant improvements in physiological markers. As these two sets of conditions have overlapping biomarkers and risk factors, we list jointly a host of positive changes. These include lowering of diastolic blood pressure, reductions in high density lipoprotein (HDL) cholesterol and triglycerides, as well as reductions in heart rate, respiratory rate, waist circumference, HbA1c and insulin resistance. A more recent review of 12 studies provided further support for these findings and also reported improvements in body mass index, quality of life and pulmonary function for both the general population and high-risk groups. Additionally, yoga has been shown to have ancillary benefits for populations at risk of cardiovascular disease and Type 2 diabetes, including stress and anxiety, better sleep and improved diet.

Yoga for Improved Mental Health

The UK was facing a severe mental health challenge even before the coronavirus pandemic of 2020/21. Now the virus has left a legacy of increased mental health problems as people struggle with the aftermath of increased social isolation, fear and the effects of surviving infection by Covid-19. A study of 402 patients hospitalized by Covid in Italy found that more than half were suffering from a psychiatric disorder a month after being discharged; 28% had post-traumatic stress disorder (PTSD), 31% had depression and 42% were suffering anxiety. The findings, published in the journal *Brain, Behavior and Immunity* in August 2020, found that, additionally, 40% of patients had interrupted sleep and 20% had symptoms of obsessive-compulsive disorder (Graham, 2020).

Yoga has been found to have robust effects on lowering negative factors in mental wellbeing – notably, by decreasing anxiety and depression, as well as physiological markers of stress, such as blood pressure, heart rate and cortisol. A meta-analysis of 12 randomized control trials of yoga interventions for patients with depressive disorders and elevated levels of depression found reductions in the severity of depression compared to receiving standard care only (Cramer *et al.*, 2018). A similar meta-analysis of 19 studies by Brinsley *et al.* (2019) reached a similar conclusion. In 2021 a study in the prestigious medical journal *JAMA Psychiatry* investigating the efficacy of yoga for generalized anxiety disorder (GAD) compared yoga with cognitive behavioural therapy (CBT); yoga was almost as effective as CBT, the most common psychological treatment for GAD (Simon *et al.*, 2021). This led to calls for yoga to be included in health systems for anxiety disorders to give patients a wider range of options.

There is increasing evidence that yoga helps to balance the autonomic nervous system (ANS). The ANS moves like a pendulum, swinging first towards the sympathetic nervous system (SNS) mobilizing energy and the fight and flight response, and then swinging back to the parasympathetic nervous system (PNS) to rest, digest and rebuild. In many chronic conditions, whether mental or physical, there is overactivity of the sympathetic system and underactivity of the parasympathetic system. In mental health conditions, this may manifest as anxiety states with an inability to curb fear and downgrade stress. Yoga has been shown to increase parasympathetic activation and rebalance the overall flexibility between these two interrelated systems (Mason and Birch, 2018). This balance is correlated with greater psychological, cognitive and even cardiovascular flexibility. Likewise, a growing collection of research reports that yoga practice in normally or excessively stressed non-practitioners or beginners is associated with a reduction of chronic levels of cortisol. Colloquially known as the stress hormone, cortisol helps us to rouse energy. However, overaction of the hypothalamic-pituitary-adrenal (HPA) axis, which releases cortisol, leads to elevated cortisol. High levels of cortisol place strain on the cardiovascular, renal, immune and nervous systems to name just a few. By both reducing stress reactivity and regulating the HPA axis, yoga is able to curtail this tendency (Riley and Park, 2015).

Possibly some of the most exciting research regarding yoga and mood regulation was conducted by Dr Chris Streeter. Gamma-aminobutyric acid (GABA), the primary inhibitory neurotransmitter in the central nervous system, helps to inhibit fear responses. GABA is notably low in various mental health conditions, from anxiety and depression, to PTSD and chronic pain, and Dr Streeter investigated the influence of yoga on this network. In a series of trials on the GABA network, Dr Streeter discovered that yoga increases GABA levels, that yoga increases GABA more than metabolically matched exercise and yoga increases GABA in those with depression (Streeter *et al.*, 2007, 2010, 2020).

Yoga to Reduce Feelings of Social Isolation

A small but growing number of studies have investigated the effects of yoga on social health, in both the general population and high-risk groups. Findings suggest that yoga creates a sense of community for those who practise it, both practically and emotionally, as participants report meeting new friends and feeling like they belong (Kishida, Mogle and Elavsky, 2019).

Additionally, yoga may improve existing interpersonal relation-ships by leading to changes in attitudes and perspective, including improving patience, kindness or self-awareness.

There are also several studies showing benefits to a specially created yoga protocol or a tailored yoga practice. Significant examples of this (two from the UK and two from the US) are given here.

- The Yoga for Healthy Lower Backs organization showed that yoga can be an effective treatment for chronic lower back pain. The research conducted by the University of York and Arthritis Research UK led to approval for the intervention by the National Institute for Health and Care Excellence (NICE) in the UK (Tilbrook *et al.*, 2011).

- NHS staff with lower back pain who were given a yoga programme took only two days off sick, compared with 43 days for staff in the control group (Hartfiel, 2014).

- A study of employees at Aetna Insurance in the US in 2011 found that employees in a yoga group dropped their stress levels by 28%, and $3,000 per employee was saved in healthcare costs per year (Goguen-Hughes, 2021).

- A pilot-level randomized control trial among nurses using yoga to improve self-care and reduce burnout showed statistically significant increases in self-care and mindfulness and a drop in emotional exhaustion (Alexander, 2015). In August 2020, a study of 18 US paediatricians found that a six-week yoga programme (called RISE) "revealed statistically significant improvements in burnout, professional fulfillment...stress, resilience, anxiety, and depression" (Scheid *et al.*, 2020, p.560). This was followed up with a study of 44 resident doctors at Harvard medical centres, showing improvement in multiple measures of psychological health (Loewenthal *et al.*, 2021).

REFERENCES

Alexander, K. R. (2015). 'Yoga for self-care and burnout prevention among nurses.' *Sage Journals. Workplace Health and Safety 63*, 10, 462–470.

Brinsley, J., Schuch, F., Lederman, O., Girard, D., *et al.* (2019). 'Effects of yoga on depressive symptoms in people with mental disorders: A systematic review and meta-analysis.' *British Journal of Sports Medicine 55*, 17, 992–1000.

Centers for Disease Control and Prevention (2021a). *What Are the Risk Factors for Lung Cancer?* Accessed on 15/10/2021 at: https://fsi.stanford.edu/news/non-communical-disease-could-cost-47-trillion-2030#:~:text=The%20United%20Nations%20has%20estimated%20that%20on%20top,trillion%20by%202030%20if%20things%20remain%20status%20quo.

Centers for Disease Control and Prevention (2021b). *Fast Facts*. Accessed on 8/9/2021 at: www.cdc.gov/tobacco/data_statistics/fact_sheets/fast_facts/index.htm.

Cramer, H., Lauche, R., Anheyer, D., Pilkington, K., *et al.* (2018). 'Yoga for anxiety: A systematic review and meta-analysis of randomized controlled trials.' *Depression and Anxiety*, 830–843.

Duff-Brown, B. (2017). *Non-Communicable Disease Could Cost $47 Trillion by 2030.* Accessed on 15/10/2021 at: https://fsi.stanford.edu/news/non-communical-disease-could-cost-47-trillion-2030#:~:text=The%20United%20Nations%20has%20estimated%20that%20on%20top,trillion%20by%202030%20if%20things%20remain%20status%20quo.

Feuerstein, G. (2001). *The Yoga Tradition: Its History, Literature, Philosophy and Practice.* Prescott, AZ: Hohm Press.

Goguen-Hughes, L. (2021). *Aetna Employees Being Mindful.* Accessed on 8/9/2021 at: www.mindful.org/aetna-employees-being-mindful.

Goldberg, E. (2016). *The Path of Modern Yoga.* Rochester, VT: Inner Traditions.

Graham, K. (2020). *Study Finds 55% of Covid-19 Survivors Suffer Mental Disorders.* Accessed on 15/10/2021 at: www.digitaljournal.com/life/study-finds-55-of-covid-19-survivors-suffer-mental-disorders/article/575916.

Hartfiel, N. (2014). 'The cost-effectiveness of yoga for preventing and reducing back pain at work: Trial protocol.' *Journal of Yoga and Physical Therapy.* DOI 10.4172/2157-7595.1000161.

Harvard Medical School (2021). *Introduction to Yoga.* Accessed on 8/9/2021 at: www.health.harvard.edu/exercise-and-fitness/introduction-to-yoga-copy.

IARC (2021). *EPIC Study Highlights.* Accessed on 8/9/2021 at: https://epic.iarc.fr/highlights/highlights.php.

Khalsa, S. B. S. (2020). *Yoga: Understanding the Biomedical Science and Research.* Accessed on 15/10/2021 at: www.youtube.com/watch?v=5w5d8IhsTCs&t=1951s.

Khalsa, S. B. S., Cohen, L., McCall, T. and Telles, S. (2016). *The Principles and Practice of Yoga in Health Care.* Pencaitland: Handspring Publishing.

Kishida, M., Mogle, J. and Elavsky, S. (2019). 'The daily influences of yoga on relational outcomes off of the mat.' *International Journal of Yoga 12*, 2, 103–113.

Loewenthal, J., Dyer, N. L., Lipsyc-Sharf, M., Borden, S., *et al.* (2021). 'Evaluation of a yoga-based mind-body intervention for resident physicians: A randomized clinical trial.' *Global Advances in Health and Medicine*, 10.1177.

Mallinson, J. and Singleton, M. (2017). 'Roots of Modern Yoga.' In *Roots of Yoga.* London: Penguin.

Mason, H. and Birch, K. (2018). *Yoga for Mental Health.* Pencaitland: Handspring Publishing.

Muktibodhnananda, S. (1998). *Hatha Yoga Pradipika.* Bihar: Bihar School of Yoga.

NCD Alliance (2021). *NCDs in the 2030 Agenda.* Accessed on 8/9/2021 at: https://ncdalliance.org/what-we-do/global-advocacy/ncds-in-2030-Agenda.

NHS Digital (2019). *Statistics on Obesity, Physical Activity and Diet, England.* Accessed on 8/9/2021 at: https://digital.nhs.uk/data-and-information/publications/statistical/statistics-on-obesity-physical-activity-and-diet/statistics-on-obesity-physical-activity-and-diet-england-2019/part-1-obesity-related-hospital-admissions.

Ornish, D. (2019). *UnDo It!* New York: Ballantine Books, Random House.

Public Health England (2021). *Obesity Profile.* Accessed on 15/10/2021 at: https://fingertips.phe.org.uk/profile/national-child-measurement-programme.

Riley, K. E. and Park, C. L. (2015). 'How does yoga reduce stress? A systematic review of mechanisms of change and guide to future inquiry.' *Health Psychology Review 9*, 3, 379–396.

Ritchie, H. and Roser, M. (2018). *Causes of Death.* Published online at OurWorldInData.org. Accessed on 15/10/2021 at: https://ourworldindata.org/causes-of-death.

Roser, M. and Ritchie, H. (2021). *Burden of Disease.* Accessed on 8/9/2021 at: https://ourworldindata.org/burden-of-disease.

Scheid, A., Dyer, N. L., Dusek, J. A. and Khalsa, S. B. S. (2020). 'A yoga-based program decreases physician burnout.' *Workplace Health and Safety*, 560–566.

Simon, N. M., Hofmann, S. G., Rosenfield, D., Hoeppner, S. S., *et al.* (2021). 'Efficacy of yoga vs cognitive behavioral therapy vs stress education for the treatment of generalized anxiety disorder: A randomized clinical trial.' *JAMA Psychiatry 78*, 1, 13–20.

Streeter, C. C., Gerbarg, P. L., Brown, R. P., Scott, T. M., *et al.* (2020). 'Thalamic gamma aminobutyric acid level changes in major depressive disorder after a 12-week Iyengar yoga and coherent breathing intervention.' *Journal of Alternative and Complementary Medicine 26*, 3, 190–197.

Streeter, C. C., Jensen, J. E., Perlmutter, R. M., Cabral, H. J., *et al.* (2007). 'Yoga asana sessions increase brain GABA levels: A pilot study.' *Journal of Alternative and Complementary Medicine 13*, 4, 419–426.

Streeter, C. C., Whitfield, T. H., Owen, L., Rein, T., *et al.* (2010). 'Effects of yoga versus walking on mood, anxiety, and brain GABA levels: A randomized controlled MRS study.' *Journal of Alternative and Complementary Medicine 16*, 11, 1145–1152.

The Good Body (2020). *38 Yoga Statistics: Discover Its (Ever-increasing) Popularity.* Accessed on 15/10/2021 at: www.thegoodbody.com/yoga-statistics.

The King's Fund (2021) *Long Term Conditions and Multi Morbidity.* Accessed on 8/9/2021 at: www.kingsfund.org.uk/projects/time-think-differently/trends-disease-and-disability-long-term-conditions-multi-morbidity.

Tilbrook, H. E., Cox, H., Hewitt, C. E., Kang'ombe, A. R., *et al.* (2011). 'Yoga for chronic low back pain: A randomized trial.' *Annals of Internal Medicine 155*, 9, 569–578.

Wellness Creative Co (2021). *Yoga Industry Growth, Market Trends & Analysis 2021.* Accessed on 15/10/2021 at: www.wellnesscreatives.com/yoga-industry-trends.

WHO (2021). *Obesity and Overweight.* Accessed on 15/10/2021 at: www.who.int/news-room/fact-sheets/detail/obesity-and-overweight.

Zuckerman, A. (2020). *Significant Yoga Statistics: 2020/2021 Benefits, Facts & Trends.* Accessed on 15/10/2021 at: https://comparecamp.com/yoga-statistics.

CHAPTER 1

The Social-Prescribing Revolution

Social prescribing is as old as the hills.

Dr Michael Dixon OBE

Imagine if everyone involved in health, social care and wellbeing in our communities pulled together to support people to be as healthy and well as possible. Imagine if visits to the family doctor were not just about health problems that had arisen, but also a conversation about opportunities to be supported in a shared enterprise of health creation for the individual and the local community.

This vision of society recognizes that many factors impact a person's health, and that medication or the surgeon's knife is not always best for an individual. In the UK, an institutional paradigm shift in this direction is taking place in the NHS. The intention is to put the patient at the centre of a more holistic vision of healthcare based around "universal personalised care". This is person-centred care, with the individual at the centre of everything and co-creating with health professionals and others their own individualized pathway to better health.

Although this vision will take time to become embedded in the culture of all GP practices (UK family doctors), policy makers see this approach as an important element in making health services sustainable. Universal personalised care makes use of "community capital" to support health. This is where social prescribing comes in.

WHAT IS SOCIAL PRESCRIBING?

In the 12 months up to October 2018, there were 307 million patient appointments in general practice in England (NHS Digital, 2018). It was reported at the 3rd International Social Prescribing Network Conference in March 2021 that in some deprived areas of the UK, up to half of all patients sought appointments for what was primarily a social problem.

Social problems leading to ill health cover a broad spectrum, including loneliness. A meta-analysis of the impact of social isolation on health found that it raised the risk of mortality to a level comparable to smoking and alcohol consumption (Holt-Lunstad, Smith and Layton, 2010). Humans are innately social creatures; when we feel we do not belong, it has consequences for our health. People with feelings of being disconnected tend towards poor diet and sedentariness. Although both issues may link to disease, they are not directly biomedical in nature and may be better dealt with by social solutions, rather than medical prescription. It can be frustrating for doctors when they see patients with problems rooted in social disconnection, as they can feel they have little to offer. It can also be a waste of precious healthcare resources.

A 2019 study of more than 21,000 people in Switzerland found that social isolation was strongly associated with poor health and behaviours that did not support health across all age groups (Hammig, 2019).

The Centers for Disease Control and Prevention in the US says social isolation significantly increases a person's risk of premature death from all causes, and that this risk may be similar to smoking, obesity and physical inactivity. It says social isolation is associated with a 50% increased risk of dementia, and that poor social relationships are also associated with a 29% increased risk of heart disease and a 32% increased risk of stroke. Furthermore, loneliness is associated with higher rates of depression, anxiety and suicide. It says loneliness among heart failure patients is associated with a near four-fold increased risk of death, a 68% increased risk of hospitalization, and a 57% increased risk of emergency department visits (Centers for Disease Control and Prevention, 2021).

There is a growing recognition of the social and economic cost of social isolation. This led the UK to appoint a Minister for Loneliness, who is directed to deal with the many social, health and political problems born from isolation.

Addressing social isolation means building up community assets that provide structures for people to engage with each other in activities that create a sense of connection and purpose, and that improve health. These features are at the heart of social prescribing. Dr Zoe Williams, TV presenter and GP, tells the story of one of her patients about whom she was concerned because she had not collected any medication for six months. The patient, Barbara, was widowed, lonely and anxious about becoming incapacitated by dementia. After several days of being unable to contact Barbara by phone, Dr Williams found that she had joined an outdoor fitness class (Silverfit) and group to learn cheerleading! Barbara had not been in for her medication because she had become active and was feeling healthy and well.

The impetus for Barbara to become more active and engage socially had come from Dr Williams, who had forgotten that she had recommended Silverfit in the first place. As Dr Williams says, social prescribing has the potential to ease the pressure on GPs by formally recognizing that patients may need a social prescription as well as a medical prescription (Williams, 2018).

The Royal College of General Practitioners (2021), in guidance to family doctors on how to ease their workload, has highlighted that social-prescribing programmes can reduce demand for GP services by up to 28%. NHS patients who are socially isolated or have a social root to their health problems can be referred to social-prescription services, enabling GPs to work more efficiently. Sometimes patients will see both their doctor and the social prescriber, and sometimes only the social prescriber. It is an approach that can make the health system run more efficiently and effectively.

A case study of a GP practice at Brownlow Health/Princes Park Health Centre in Liverpool, which introduced social prescribing in March 2019, found that it had a significant impact on the number of patient appointments. In this case, the surgery's receptionist became the social prescriber and saw 40 patients over a three-month period. Three of the patients had seen their doctor a total of 20 times during the 10 months before the new system was put in place. During the three months that the patients saw the social prescriber, there was only one GP appointment by one of the patients (NHS England, 2021a).

In January 2019, NHS England issued its mandate and goals for the next ten years. The *NHS Long Term Plan* (NHS England, 2019a) expressed the importance of community health and the benefits of social prescribing. The Secretary of State for Health and Social Care allocated £500 million to support social prescribing, embedding the movement in the official culture of UK healthcare.

The *NHS Long Term Plan* describes social prescribing as:

> Helping people to use services in their community to improve their health and wellbeing – this could be something like a cookery group run by a local charity. (NHS England, 2019b)

The Healthy London Partnership, supported by the Mayor of London, NHS England, London Councils and Public Health England, defines social prescribing as:

> ...a way of linking patients in primary care with sources of support within the community. It provides GPs with a non-medical referral option that can operate alongside existing treatments to improve health and wellbeing. (Healthy London Partnership, n.d., p.1)

The NHS sees social prescribing aligning with and complementing its roll-out of a comprehensive model of "personalised care". This model sees health and social care working closely together to give patients an individualized package of care. The aspiration is to have 2.5 million NHS patients in England receiving personalised care by 2023/24. This will include the spread of "Personal Care Budgets", which will give patients some control over how money on their health and social care is spent.

UNIVERSAL PERSONALISED CARE

Health service leaders have emphasized the importance of personalised care:

> Personalised Care and Support Planning is key for people receiving health and social care services. It is an essential tool to integrate the person's experience of all the services they access so that they have one joined-up plan that covers their health and wellbeing needs. (NHS England, 2021b)

Integrating health, social care, personalised care and social prescribing is partly an attempt to support patients to make the mental shift towards taking more responsibility for their health and wellbeing, and to give patients more control over their health. For example, a patient requiring the support of a carer at home would have more choice over which agency provided that care, and they might choose a local person they know to become their paid carer. Personal Care Budgets could also become a potential source of income for those offering social-prescribing services, which patients may choose to purchase.

However, in these early years of the social-prescribing movement, NHS funding is being largely restricted to employing Social Prescribing Link Workers who become part of the GP practice/Primary Care Network (PCN) team and receive patient referrals directly from GPs, nurses and (increasingly) skilled-up reception workers who can intercept patients who need a social prescription before they unnecessarily occupy a GP appointment.

LINK WORKERS – AN EMERGING PROFESSION

Under the *NHS Long Term Plan*, over 1000 Social Prescribing Link Workers have already been employed by PCNs across England (similar appointments are taking place in Scotland, Wales and Northern Ireland) (NHS England, 2019a).

You may already be aware of, or have met, a Social Prescribing Link Worker (sometimes called Social Navigators or Community Connectors). It is their job to become aware of all the social-prescribing opportunities and resources in the communities they serve. A Link Worker will commonly have a caseload of patients deemed to have social rather than medical problems. Over the course of six to ten one-hour sessions, they will work with the patient to co-create an appropriate social prescription that meets their needs.

For example, a patient with drug or alcohol dependency problems may be supported by the Link Worker to join an appropriate addiction counselling programme. Someone with debt problems could be helped to receive support from Citizens Advice or a debt-management bureau. Many of these services have been around for decades. The difference is that the Link Worker provides a point of support for the clients that interlinks with their healthcare and acts as a joined-up solution to their problems. Link Workers may support their clients over several months to go through a process that leads to change and hopefully a resolution. Whereas a client with social problems might have been referred to an external agency, the process is now overseen by their Link Worker and records of each social prescription are included on patient records.

Many Link Workers are members of the National Association of Link Workers (NALW), which acts as a professional body and provides training, professional guidance, resources and shared practice via networking events. YIHA recognized early on that Link Workers would become key people connecting patients to the Yoga4Health/Yoga on Prescription social-prescribing ten-week programme. YIHA was a sponsor for the first NALW national conference for Link Workers held in London during 2019.

Link Workers have little, if any, budget for the activities they offer clients and will usually be accessing free programmes. The absence of significant direct investment into social-prescribing activities is a challenge for the future. This picture may change as further research in the field of health economics builds on existing data showing the cost-benefit analysis of social prescribing – potentially saving tens of millions of pounds in direct healthcare costs down the line. In the meantime, the NHS and others continue to rely heavily on charities to provide activities, and on volunteers whose services may already be overstretched. This means that for some social-prescribing programmes, it may be unavoidable to ask patients to contribute to the cost of their social prescription.

PATIENT ACTIVATION

Society has moved away from the traditional and paternalistic "doctor knows best" attitude, in which patients passively received a diagnosis and prescription from their GP and unquestioningly did what they were told. This model disempowered patients and did little to account for the influence of lifestyle on health.

Patient-centred care is informed by an evidence base and clinical judgements, alongside listening and an empathetic approach to health. This places a new mandate on professionals to embrace shared decision-making. They not only discuss options with patients, but also understand patients' priorities, needs, motivations and choices (which may include no treatment) and align health plans with all this in mind. This shift in the model of health both empowers patients and places responsibility for their wellbeing back on their shoulders, at least partially.

The aforementioned Dr Michael Dixon is a pioneer in social prescribing, and the current Chair of the College of Medicine and Integrated Health.

Perhaps it was the philosophy and psychology he studied at the University of Oxford before training as a doctor at Guy's Hospital in London that gave him the breadth of vision to see beyond orthodox approaches to medicine. Since 2007, he and his GP partners at their practice in Devon, England, have run the Culm Valley Integrated Centre for Health. Through years of experience, he has crafted a vision and a model for the future of general practice by pioneering prevention and treating patients holistically. The practice makes use of complementary therapies – including yoga. The approach caught the eye of Prince Charles and gained his approval.

In the sense that people have intuitively recognized the social aspects of health since time immemorial, social prescribing is, as Dr Dixon says, "as old as the hills" (Dixon, 2021). However, in 2015, all the work and initiatives in this area was pulled together under one roof when Dr Dixon co-founded the National Social Prescribing Steering Group with Dr Marie Polley.

This led to the creation of the National Social Prescribing Network at its inaugural conference in London in January 2016, co-funded by the University of Westminster, the Wellcome Trust and the Fit for Work UK coalition. The event was supported by the College of Medicine and Integrated Health.

SOCIAL PRESCRIBING – A BRIGHT FUTURE

Our optimism about the future for social prescribing is based partly on how far and how fast the UK has come in such a short time. The January 2016 inaugural conference on social prescribing produced a seminal report that defined the landscape of social prescribing. It is worth reflecting on a short excerpt from the report:

Social prescribing acknowledges the need for patients to access non-clinical resources to enable them to improve their health and wellbeing. This approach also recognises that a large proportion of health outcomes are the result of the social and economic determinants of health, not just the quality of the healthcare that individuals receive. Health is no longer about the absence of disease. Today, the challenge we face is to create a system within which people are able to adapt, change and self-manage in the face of social, physical and emotional challenges.

Whilst healthcare professionals are best placed to support patients' clinical needs, they are not always equipped to help patients with their social and economic issues which also have an important impact on their health. Social prescribing offers patients the opportunity and, crucially, the time to talk about their issues in an informal and often non-clinical setting. The link worker aims to increase levels of patient activation, motivation and self-efficacy through discussion, coaching and goal setting with the patient – often seeing patients several times to review their individual goals. Link workers may also suggest appropriate resources and support for the patient to access depending on their specific needs. The aim is to provide the patient with a 'voice' in this process. These resources may be within the GP practice or via voluntary or community groups, or created, designed and maintained by the social prescribing organisation.

Using a social prescribing approach facilitates appropriate care and widens the scope of what is possible to do as a community of health practitioners. Social prescribing has started to connect the many, and often disconnected, organisations working across a geographical area, a locality, or a neighbourhood. In the narrowest sense, social prescribing acts as a signposting service to the available local resources. In its broadest sense, social prescribing may connect the GP practice, the voluntary groups, the services designed by the social prescribing organisations, the housing provider, the children's centre, the timebank, the faith organisations, the police and so on. (Social Prescribing Network, 2016, p.9)

The Benefits of Social Prescribing

Physical and emotional health and wellbeing	Cost effectiveness and sustainability	Builds up local community
Improve resilience Self-confidence Self-esteem Improve modifiable lifestyle factors Improve mental health Improve quality of life	Prevention Reduction in frequent primary care use Savings across the care pathway Reduced prescribing of medicines	Increases awareness of what is available Stronger links between voluntary and healthcare sectors Community resilience Nurture community assets
Behaviour change Lifestyle Sustained change Ability to self-care Autonomy Activation Motivation Learning new skills	**Capacity to build up the voluntary sector** More volunteering Volunteer graduates running schemes Addressing unmet needs of patients Enhance social infrastructure	**Social determinants of ill health** Better employability Reduce isolation Social welfare law advice Reach marginalized groups Increase skills

Social Prescribing Network, 2016

This report generated greater momentum within the social-prescribing movement to become what Dr Marie Anne Essam – a Clinical Lead and Ambassador for Social Prescribing – described as "the most transformative and fabulous treatment I have had to offer my patients in 30 years" (Essam, 2019).

On 23 October 2019 England's Secretary of State for Health and Social Care launched the National Academy for Social Prescribing. The academy has a multimillion-pound budget directed towards forging partnerships across various sectors including the arts, health, sports, leisure and the natural environment within the social-prescribing space to promote health and wellbeing at a national and local level. It also aims to champion social prescribing and the work of local communities in connecting people within the wellbeing arena.

The inclusion for the first time of social prescribing as a main plank in the *NHS Long Term Plan* means that the time is ripe for this movement to become embedded in healthcare. Britain is leading the world in this field, with bodies like the College of Medicine and Integrated Health providing leadership, including its manifesto for change (College of Medicine and Integrated Health, 2021). In the coming years, there is an opportunity to step into a new healthier world of self-care and community.

THE COVID-19 PANDEMIC
Healthcare systems have been stretched to breaking point by the Covid-19 pandemic. Many of those worst affected were more vulnerable because of underlying lifestyle-related diseases, leading to extra pressure on already overstretched systems. An infectious disease pandemic has exposed the importance of self-led care for those with NCDs who were among the most at-risk groups. The situation was exacerbated by lockdown and social distancing, leading to the worst crisis of social isolation that we have ever seen globally. When social prescribing was conceived, no one knew how vital this scheme would be. As we move forward into a period of recovery, social prescribing is likely to become ever-more important. Within this purview, yoga offers a practice that not only keeps individuals connected to each other, but also bestows health and fosters a sense of connection with Self when other resources may not be available. YIHA recently co-sponsored a conference to focus on the importance of yoga in healthcare after the pandemic with social prescribing at centre stage. Yoga can play an important role in the social-prescribing movement, as we discover in the next chapter.

REFERENCES
Centers for Disease Control and Prevention (2021). *Alzheimer's Disease and Healthy Aging: Loneliness and Social Isolation Linked to Serious Health Conditions*. Accessed on 9/9/2021 at: www.cdc.gov/aging/publications/features/lonely-older-adults.html.
College of Medicine and Integrated Health (2021). *Manifesto*. Accessed on 9/9/2021 at: https://collegeofmedicine.org.uk/tag/manifesto.
Dixon, M. (2021). *Address to the Third International Social Prescribing Network Conference*. 4–5 March 2021.
Essam, M. A. (2019). *National Association of Link Workers Annual Conference*. 8 July 2019.
Hammig, O. (2019). 'Health risks associated with social isolation in general and in young, middle and old age.' *PLOS ONE 14*, 7.
Healthy London Partnership (n.d.). *Health Committee Meeting: Social Prescribing in London, Appendix*. Accessed on 15/10/2021 at: www.london.gov.uk/about-us/londonassembly/meetings/documents/s73422/05a%20SPscopingpaper.pdf.

Holt-Lunstad, J., Smith, T. B. and Layton, J. B. (2010). 'Social relationships and mortality risk: A meta-analytic review.' *PLOS Medicine 7, 7*, e1000316.

NHS Digital (2018). *Appointments in General Practice.* Accessed on 9/9/2021 at: https://digital.nhs.uk/data-and-information/publications/statistical/appointments-in-general-practice/oct-2018.

NHS England (2019a). *NHS Long Term Plan.* Accessed on 9/9/2021 at: www.long termplan.nhs.uk.

NHS England (2019b). *NHS Long Term Plan Easy Read.* Accessed on 15/10/2021 at: www. longtermplan.nhs.uk/wp-content/uploads/2019/01/easy-read-long-term-plan-v2. pdf.

NHS England (2021a). *Social Prescribing: Reducing Non-Medical GP Appointments and Delivering a Better Service for Patients – Brownlow Health @ Princes Park Health Centre, North West.* Accessed on 9/9/2021 at: www.england.nhs.uk/gp/case-studies/social-prescribing-reducing-non-medical-gp-appointments-and-delivering-a-better-service-for-patients-brownlow-health-princes-park-health-centre-north-west.

NHS England (2021b). *Personalised Care and Support Planning.* Accessed on 9/9/2021 at: www.england.nhs.uk/ourwork/patient-participation/patient-centred/planning.

Royal College of General Practitioners (2021). *The 10 High Impact Actions.* Accessed on 9/9/2021 at: www.rcgp.org.uk/-/media/Files/Primary-Care-Development/RCGP-spotlight-on-the-10-high-impact-actions-may-2018.ashx?la=en.

Social Prescribing Network (2016). *Report of the Annual Social Prescribing Network Conference.* Accessed on 15/10/2021 at: www.artshealthresources.org.uk/wp-content/uploads/2017/01/2016-Social-Prescribing-Network-First-Conference-Report.pdf.

Williams, Z. (2018). *The King's Fund Social Prescribing Seminar.* 20 November 2018.

CHAPTER 2

Yoga on Prescription – the Yoga4Health Protocol

Yoga is the settling of the agitations of the mind.

Yoga Sutras of Patanjali

In early 2017, YIHA was contacted by the NHS West London Clinical Commissioning Group (CCG) and asked to create a yoga social-prescribing programme. West London CCG had become aware of YIHA's mission to integrate yoga in UK healthcare using evidence-based methods and well-trained teachers with high professional standards.

West London CCG (which no longer exists due to NHS reorganization) was well-known as a pioneer in the field of social prescribing and offered its NHS patients an impressive range of non-medical support for their health needs. Under the leadership of the then Chair of the CCG, Dr Fiona Butler, and Self Care and Third Sector Commissioning Manager, Kalwant Sahota, a decision was taken to introduce a yoga social-prescribing programme. One of the hopes was to evaluate the effectiveness of a yoga social-prescribing programme and develop a model that others might use to deliver yoga in a safe and effective way.

Over the course of the following six months, YIHA developed a ten-week evidence-based protocol, designed to promote self-care skills and bring about positive lifestyle change. The core of the protocol was created by the authors of this book, Heather Mason, founder of The Minded Institute, and Paul Fox, former Chair of The British Wheel of Yoga and a YIHA board member. A range of leading experts were involved to develop and refine the protocol, including Dr Robin Monro, the founder of the UK yoga therapy profession, Dr Sat Bir Singh Khalsa from Harvard Medical School, Emily Brett, the founder of Ourmala, Dr Ned Hartfiel from Bangor University, Alison Trewhela from Yoga for Healthy Lower Backs and leading yoga therapist Lisa Kaley-Isley.

The Yoga on Prescription Yoga4Health protocol was designed as an early intervention programme to be delivered to patients at risk of developing chronic diseases or more serious mental health conditions. It was important to YIHA that its Yoga4Health teachers would be able to form cohorts of 12–15 patients and teach them in a group setting with appropriate modifications. This group format was pivotal to it being a social-prescribing intervention. The target patients presented with the following health needs and could be placed in the same group.

- Those at risk of cardiovascular disease with a QRISK score of 10 (derived from a series of questions about health, habits and family history, and sometimes followed up by blood tests), suggesting that based on the current evidence, this individual was at a certain percentage of risk of a cardiac event, such as a heart attack or stroke, within the next ten years.

- Those diagnosed as being pre-diabetic and therefore at risk of developing Type 2 diabetes. Often this would be associated with a patient being overweight or obese, not taking enough exercise and possibly smoking. Lifestyle and blood test results would typically alert the GP practice that a patient had fallen into this category.

- Those suffering stress or mild to moderate anxiety and/or depression.

- Those experiencing social isolation.

These referral criteria were chosen because they encapsulate a broad base of individuals with growing health needs, where lifestyle is a significant factor in the presentation. By supporting behavioural change via yoga, it was hypothesized that patients' health trajectories might change, reducing pressure on the health services and improving individual quality of life.

An intervention at early stages presented the opportunity to work with a broad spectrum of patients and allowed the programme designers to include groups with some of the most common health problems, which could require significant healthcare resources in the future if left unchecked. Unlike patients with more serious illnesses or various co-morbidities requiring much more specific yogic practices, the patients referred to Yoga4Health programmes at early stages of unwellness have shared physiological needs even though diagnosis may seem quite different.

Alongside these inclusionary criteria, and working with doctors and other health professionals, YIHA also developed exclusionary criteria. These are some of the main reasons why a patient would not be suitable for the ten-week programme. They include more severe mental health conditions, such as severe depression and anxiety, chronic psychosis or PTSD; those with anti-social behaviours; those in recent recovery from substance misuse; those receiving ongoing treatment for serious diseases like cancer or kidney disease; and those with neurocognitive decline that would compromise their ability to follow the class. Those with late-stage COPD, a recent cardiac event or acute inflammatory conditions were also excluded, as these groups need more individualized treatment. Those with lower back pain problems were additionally excluded, because the underlying causes are so variable and their unique needs require elaborate assessment for the safe practice of yoga (and we collaborate with the providers of the NICE-approved Yoga for Healthy Lower Backs programme). The exclusionary criteria included conditions that were more the purview of yoga therapists, often working one-to-one.

The protocol was successfully piloted on two cohorts of West London CCG NHS staff and evaluated by GPs, patient representatives and experts in social prescribing.

> I decided to take up yoga to get some fitness back into my life and also try to become healthier as I head towards retirement. Little did I know just how wonderful yoga is and how it would change my life. I now wish that I had discovered yoga when I was much younger – I would now be much fitter, more resilient and would have benefited from a greater sense of wellbeing much sooner, and some life skills that will be of benefit each and every day. (Melissa, NHS employee)

Researchers from the University of Westminster, led by Dr Tina Cartwright, were appointed to evaluate the programme, which was then delivered as a social-prescribing project to 279 NHS patients in the

West London CCG catchment area. Marie Polley, the Co-Chair of the Social Prescribing Network, chaired research meetings to make sure the intervention followed the written guidance for all social-prescribing programmes. However, this still allowed YIHA to modify the programme in real time occasionally to meet the needs of patients and the healthcare system. Rigorous techniques were used to gather benchmark data before patients began the ten-week programme, as well as gathering further data at the end of the programme and three months later.

YOGA4HEALTH ON SOCIAL PRESCRIPTION: A MIXED METHODS EVALUATION
Dr Tina Cartwright, Dr Rebecca Richards, Amy Edwards and Dr Anna Cheshire (2019)

Dr Cartwright and her colleagues reached the following overall conclusion:

> Patient reported outcome data demonstrated significant improvements from baseline to post-intervention on all outcome measures, which were sustained 3 months after the Yoga4Health programme. Service users showed statistically significant and clinically meaningful decreases in perceived stress, anxiety, and depression suggesting the mental health benefits of the course. Significant improvements were also found for patient activation (confidence in managing one's health), wellbeing and social connectedness, highlighting the programme's positive psychological and social benefits. (p.6)

The analysis further found that:

> Cost data showed that for every £1 spent on Yoga4Health there was a ROI of £2.19, mostly accruing due to a reduction in health service usage. (p.7)

The full evaluation is available via the YIHA website and the University of Westminster.[1] Here we provide a summary.

---

1   https://westminsterresearch.westminster.ac.uk/item/qz6v1/yoga4health-on-social-prescription-a-mixed-methods-evaluation#:~:text=Yoga4Health%20on%20social%20prescription%3A%20a%20mixed%20methods%20evaluation,with%20ROI_final_.p%20...%20%201%20more%20rows%20

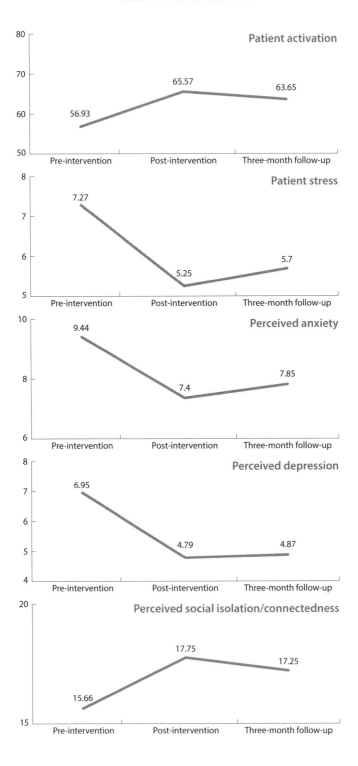

Key Findings

- Patient Activation Measure (PAM) went up significantly for 62% of patients.

- Stress as measured by the PSS-4 scale was significantly down.

- Depression as measured by the HADS scale was significantly reduced.

- Social connectedness as measured by the HFS scale was significantly increased.

- Sense of wellbeing, including life satisfaction, purpose and happiness, was up. Anxiety rates fell.

- Physical health also showed meaningful improvements, with 45% of patients reporting better health, and waist circumference reduced by an average of 14 cm.

Patients either self-referred to the programme or were referred by their GP. Of the 365 service users booked on the Yoga4Health programme, 279 attended at least one of the ten sessions, which were run over a total of 22 courses between February 2018 and May 2019. The patients were predominately female (83%), 44% were educated to degree level, 40% identified as Black, Asian and minority ethnic (BAME) and 48% rated their health as poor or fair at baseline. Their primary motivations for attending the programme were: 1) improve their psychological health; 2) improve their physicality, such as flexibility, balance or fitness; 3) improve or maintain their physical health and wellbeing.

Mental Health

Patients entering the Yoga4Health programme had above average scores for perceived stress. Their average score of 7.27 (on the PSS-4 scale) fell to 5.25 by the end of the course. Average stress in the UK population is 5.56 for men and 6.38 for women.

Anxiety and depression HADS scores showed that 51% of patients experienced a statistically meaningful improvement in their anxiety, and 50% a statistically meaningful improvement in their depression.

Overall, the Yoga4Health course decreased ratings of social isolation and increased service users' sense of connection with others. (p.24)

The breathing exercises were reported to be the most useful component of the course due to their application to everyday life... Service users thus appeared to have developed a toolkit to manage issues in their daily lives. (p.27)

I have learnt to breathe properly and to use this mechanism to combat my stress levels...that moment of stress will pass and life goes on. (p.27, patient response in follow-up questionnaire and focus group)

I have continued to feel more relaxed, able to deal with stress better and maintain a positive attitude. (p.27, patient response in follow-up questionnaire and focus group)

Physical Health

In total, 45% of patients reported that their perceived physical health had improved by at least one level. The number identifying their health as poor fell from 11% to 5%, while those reporting very good health rose from 8% to 17% (18% at three-month follow-up).

Overall, 80% of patients reported improvements in their stress levels, mental health and physical health.

When I have a specific pain or injury, I now know which are the best poses and stretches to do. (p.29)

I go to three yoga classes a week now...when they stopped over Christmas for two weeks, my body practically seized up, I got really stiff. (p.29, patient response in follow-up questionnaire and focus group)

My insomnia is almost gone. (p.29, patient response in follow-up questionnaire and focus group)

Diet and Nutrition

Patients reported to the researchers that they had become more aware of their eating habits and were able to change to healthier habits by reducing junk food and increasing fruit and vegetable consumption.

There's no point in going to yoga and then going and having spaghetti bolognese and three cakes and so it made you more aware of your body and what you were eating and how you were living. I genuinely believe that. (p.29, patient focus group)

Enjoyment

Patients reported high levels of enjoyment of the course, giving an average rating of 6.36 out of 7. Although the sample is slightly biased towards those who completed the course, 94% had a very favourable view of their enjoyment of the yoga classes.

> Many service users cited the personalised, inclusive approach of the yoga teachers as key to their enjoyment of sessions. (p.34)

Home Practice

Three months after completing the Yoga4Health programme, patients practised yoga on average just over two days a week; 44% had begun attending a local yoga class; half used the Yoga4Health resources to continue their home practice.

The course manual containing home-practice sequences was described as very or somewhat useful by 87%. Some 74% found the home-practice videos somewhat or very helpful.

> I know how beneficial practising yoga has been/is for me so that moti-vates me to continue to practice. (p.39, patient follow-up questionnaire)

Return on Investment (ROI)

Cost data showed that for every £1 spent on Yoga4Health, there was a ROI of £2.19, mostly accruing due to a reduction in health service usage. This figure is similar to those reported by other social-prescribing schemes. It represents a ROI for only a one-year period and not lifetime savings. The Yoga4Health project unit costs were £307.76 per patient. It is important to note that this ROI involved the cost of the research, a large portion of the funding. If taught without the research, the ROI is likely to be at least a third higher.

Conclusions

The evaluation found that it is possible to effectively develop a yoga intervention for a diverse group of NHS patients that can be delivered within an NHS social prescribing pathway. (p.7)

This evaluation confirms the importance of having experienced and supported yoga teachers and a provider with local knowledge to access diverse patient groups. (p.7)

It was a very special course and I am very lucky to have been part of it. It was life changing. (p.7, patient response in follow-up questionnaire and focus group)

I wholeheartedly think it should be introduced within the NHS. I think it's about time. (p.7, patient response in follow-up questionnaire and focus group)

THE STRUCTURE OF THE YOGA4HEALTH PROTOCOL

Patients on the Yoga4Health Yoga on Prescription programme sign up for ten consecutive weeks of lifestyle change through yoga. Heather Mason developed a course model in which each session lasts two hours and is made up of the following components.

- Initial introduction and psycho-education – psycho-education was developed by Heather to provide a short sustained teaching on a particular topic, such as balancing the nervous system, reducing stress and living a healthier life – physically and mentally. Psycho-educations introduce the week's class theme: 5 minutes.

- Settling of students and breath awareness using the week's breath practice: 5 minutes.

- Yoga posture practice starting for all in a chair and moving to the mat for those who can: 70 minutes.

- Relaxation relating to the class theme: 15 minutes.

- Final breathing/*pranayama* practice: 5 minutes.

- Group discussion to share experiences of the practice and of home practice: 20 minutes.

An essential part of the Yoga4Health programme is home practice. Students are encouraged to practise every day, even if only for five to ten minutes. Studies show that a regular practice builds habit formation and behavioural change (Gardner and Rebar, 2019). Dose level studies such as the 2020 study by Dr Streeter on yoga for depression found that more practice really matters in terms of improving outcomes (Streeter *et al.*, 2020).

The YIHA programme seeks to support behavioural change by encouraging and inspiring students towards more home practice throughout the ten weeks. During the first session of the programme, all students are given an extensive student manual that includes four different home practices, with description and pictures for each week of the course. This includes long and short home-practice sequences to do on a chair or on a yoga mat, based on weekly themes. Patients are also encouraged to create an account on the YIHA website where they can then access over 40 home-practice videos (long and short chair and mat versions for each of the ten weeks of the programme) and other videos on the breathing practices covered during the ten sessions. These two options of videos and written content make the home practice more accessible, as not everyone uses online resources.

Yoga4Health teachers introduce self-care themes and self-care skills that drill home the message that a daily practice is vital to create the changes to better health that patients need. Throughout the course, patients are invited to consider all the yoga techniques they learn in class as part of their "yoga toolkit", which can be deployed in everyday situations to help them cope more skilfully with life and support their inner resilience.

To this end, all patients are given home-practice sheets to mark the days when they practise and for how long. This becomes part of YIHA's data collection – along with an initial benchmark data form and end-of-course form that Yoga4Health teachers use to collect ongoing information on the effectiveness of the Yoga on Prescription/Yoga4Health programme (in addition to the formal University of Westminster evaluation). Keeping a daily journal during an experience of transformation is a well-known technique that helps to draw out experience and make it explicit on the page. A study by researchers from the University of Rochester Medical Center (2021) found that journaling was a helpful tool in managing mental health, including stress and anxiety.

> You may have stopped using a diary once you reached adulthood. But the concept and its benefits still apply. Now it's called journaling. It's simply writing down your thoughts and feelings to understand them more clearly. And if you struggle with stress, depression, or anxiety, keeping a journal can be a great idea. It can help you gain control of your emotions and improve your mental health. (University of Rochester Medical Center, 2021)

Patients also talk about their home practice during the group feedback session. Hearing about how others fit their home practice into busy lives helps to motivate patients to maintain a daily practice and take on the new healthy habit of yoga.

We recognize that motivation is key to lifestyle change. Many patients who have completed the programme have told us that they have become devoted yoga practitioners and continue to benefit greatly in a wide range of ways, including feeling stronger, more flexible, more able to cope, less overwhelmed and more positive, and sleeping more soundly.

The organization Science of Behaviour Change is dedicated to researching the emerging field of behavioural medicine (Science of Behaviour Change, 2021). Researchers there set out to answer the simple question: why do people find it so hard to stick to a diet or exercise regime? This led them to create a conceptual framework to identify, measure and influence the key mechanisms underlying successful change in health behaviours.

One key concept developed is "temporal discounting". To what extent are patients able to ignore immediate rewards (such as unhealthy snacks) and focus instead on the larger future rewards of avoiding obesity? Thinking about future goals in a specific and detailed way is one strategy (called "episodic future thinking") to address this problem.

In the National Institutes of Health *Science of Behaviour Change Project Overview* published in 2017, Science of Behaviour Change states that "behaviours are among the most important factors that determine whether people will live long, healthy lives". It estimates that the choices humans make account for almost 40% of the risk associated with preventable premature deaths in the US (National Institutes of Health, 2017).

On the Yoga4Health programme, we aim to apply these evidence-based principles of behaviour change through our weekly theme and psycho-education. We help people find their primary wishes and motivations and consider how to connect these to everyday decisions. We educate people on the ebbs and flows of yoga practice and highlight that their challenges are not insurmountable obstacles but fodder for transformation. When coupled with the faculties naturally nourished through yoga practice, such as greater embodiment, mindfulness and connectedness – alongside some simple ideas about diet and exercise – motivation increases, preparing the ground for transformation.

The entire pathway is also set up to support change. For example, by running Yoga4Health as a GP-referral or NHS Link Worker referral, the programme benefits from the collective weight of NHS healthcare. A patient may have heard about yoga and know vaguely that it might do them some good. However, they are much more strongly motivated to try yoga by seeing Yoga4Health leaflets in the surgery waiting room, seeing a screenshot on the TV monitor advertising the start date of the next Yoga4Health course or having an NHS Link Worker advise them that this looks like the programme they need.

Doctors are becoming more aware of the need for long-term solutions for patient health, rather than short-term fixes. They will prescribe drugs for their patient who has developed Type 2 diabetes but also encourage them to exercise more and adjust their diet – pointing out that this is one disease that can be reversed by lifestyle change. By encouraging patients to take responsibility for their own health via person-centred care and self-care through activities like yoga, the health professionals we work with are supporting behaviour change. Doctors remain highly respected professionals, and patients listen to their advice. This can be motivating when overcoming short-term lifestyle habits in favour of long-term change.

During Session 1 of the Yoga4Health programme, patients are invited to take some time to reflect on what they really wish for in their life. Often, patients will know that they need to make lifestyle changes to improve their health. However, many patients will continue with lifestyle habits that put them at risk. What we seek to uncover during this time of reflection are deeper motivations capable of supporting more fundamental shifts in perspective and behaviour. Often patients may not be aware of their deeper motivations until they have undertaken this process of self-reflection.

One patient wished to visit her daughter in South Africa but did not feel well enough or resilient enough to undertake the journey. It was highly motivating for her to hold that goal in her mind during the inevitable struggles that arise in any programme of transformation and change. By tapping this vision and diligently attending the programme and home practising, she eventually felt strong enough to make the journey. Connecting patients to a compelling inner goal, which they may or may not choose to share with the group, is instrumental in inspiring positive action.

A further source of motivation is the way in which we invite Yoga-4Health patients to consider the bigger picture of the state of healthcare in the UK (and in many other countries). The relentless growth of lifestyle-related diseases (NCDs) and aging populations is placing a huge burden on health services. In the UK, there is great pride and affection for the NHS. During the Covid-19 crisis there was a "Clap for Carers" every Thursday evening for several months, when people stood outside their front doors and clapped, banged saucepans or played musical instruments in a show of solidarity with health and care workers. The feeling of doing something small for the greater good is compelling. On the programme, patients enjoy the thought that their individual lifestyle change and effort – when combined with everyone else's individual effort – could make a positive difference to the NHS by easing the burden of chronic disease.

GROUP DISCUSSION AND SOCIAL CONNECTION

The deep personal motivation that patients discover, and these other motivating factors, all feed into the group discussion lasting around 20 minutes at the end of every Yoga4Health class. This is one of the components of our programme that makes it different to a regular yoga class and helps it to align with social prescribing. Yoga students do not usually get up from relaxation and breathing to then share with the group how they felt during the practice, how that week's theme worked for them and how they are doing overall. But this is what we invite our patients to do, and it binds them in a very close-knit group, fostering social connection and motivating them.

Group support enables individual patients to feel a sense of togetherness – that they are not alone on their yoga journey. For those on the programme due to social isolation, this can be an inspiring experience of community and common purpose. Reflecting on their experiences in the patient manual after each week also supports this aspect of the programme.

Yoga cultivates self-awareness through breath and movement. When a person is completely absorbed in their practice and dwelling almost entirely in the present moment, the experience of the felt body can be vivid. However, it is still easy to float out of a yoga class, go to bed and wake up having forgotten most of what took place (nevertheless, the benefits will still be there). Through group discussion, patients articulate their experience in words and concepts that sink deeper into their conscious mind and become a resource of mind-body learning. By hearing others speak about their experiences, they also benefit from fresh perspectives and new insights that might refine their understanding of their own experience.

The group discussion becomes a time of shared learning, in which patients can receive clarification, individual instruction and further advice on modifying posture practice. Sharing takes place in a structured and orderly way, presided over by the teacher so that everyone feels supported and part of a community of practice. So strong are the bonds created that many students continue to stay connected to fellow course members when their ten-week programme ends, and some meet up to practise the Yoga4Health sequences together.

SELF-EFFICACY

As a social-prescribing programme, social bonds are at the heart of the Yoga4Health programme. The strength of these social bonds flourishes during the course. In fact, YIHA has experienced that by weeks nine and ten, patients may become concerned that their weekly gathering and social connection is about to end. Sometimes they express the sentiment: "Can our group carry on?" However, like other social-prescribing programmes, part of the remit from the NHS was to create sustainability beyond the ten sessions. Patients are prepared for the final sessions, given resources signposting them to suitable local yoga classes and reminded that they have ongoing access to the home-practice sequences as online videos or via their patient manuals.

During the final weeks of the programme, it is hoped that patients will be reaching an increased level of self-efficacy. The term "self-efficacy" was first coined in 1977 by the Canadian-American psychologist Albert Bandura, a professor at Stanford University. He defined the idea as a person's belief in their capability to exercise control over their own functioning and over events that affect their lives. High self-efficacy can provide the foundation for motivation, wellbeing and personal accomplishment (Bandura, 1997).

Self-efficacy in the context of healthcare in the UK is measured by means of the PAM – Patient Activation Measure – a simple set of questions to assess an individual's knowledge, skill and confidence in managing their health. Professor Alf Collins, Clinical Advisor to NHS England's Personalised Care Group, describes PAM as "at the heart of personalised care" (NHS England, 2021, p.3). He describes patient activation as a "light bulb moment" for doctors who had previously been puzzled by how difficult it was to engage with some patients about managing their long-term conditions (NHS England, 2021, p.3).

Many doctors and healthcare professionals access the PAM, which has become widely used in primary care. Doctors are increasingly keen to see patient PAM scores rise through prevention programmes like Yoga4Health, because a high score means that the person understands the importance of taking a proactive role in managing their health and has the skills and confidence to do so. PAM scores are not just raised by specific programmes, but by the whole culture and ethos of healthcare. Family doctors are learning to conduct consultations using the "shared decision-making" model in which patients feel they have an equal role in the decisions about their treatment.

As the University of Westminster evaluation shows, Yoga4Health increases PAM scores significantly.

YOGA4HEALTH TEACHER QUALITY

Yoga4Health teachers who take the YIHA training are among the most skilled yoga teachers in the UK. Those who take the 60-hour professional training course to deliver the Yoga4Health protocol all have high-quality yoga-teacher qualifications, have been teaching for a minimum of three years (usually it is much longer) and can demonstrate a track record of being able to meet the needs of a diverse range of students by offering modified practices. Yoga teachers who are also GPs, nurses, physiotherapists and occupational therapists, and a consultant psychiatrist, are among the health professionals who have trained to deliver the Yoga4Health protocol.

Yoga4Health teachers hold a current Disclosure and Barring Service (DBS) certificate, have undertaken Adult Safeguarding Training and first-aid training, and are fully insured. During 2021, YIHA achieved accreditation for the Yoga4Health programme from the Personalised Care Institute (PCI). The PCI was set up by the Royal College of General Practitioners and NHS England to accredit training courses in the field of social prescribing and social care, under the umbrella of universal personalised care. The course has been lengthened to 60 hours to encompass further professional training to equip yoga teachers to work in healthcare and be regarded by others as healthcare colleagues.

As part of Yoga4Health training, our teachers learn to hold a healing safe space for the patients in their class and offer an extended duty of care. This feels like a new role to many, but it highlights that they are part of something bigger than an individual yoga class or programme. They have become integrated into healthcare and are helping to address societal-level problems of lifestyle-related disease.

As they organize each ten-week programme, Yoga4Health teachers begin to build the social network that will sustain their cohort of patients. This involves communicating by email, text and telephone to every patient before the programme starts, being available for two hours each week for patients to call and, if a patient fails to attend class, contacting them to check that they are OK. This begins the process of ensuring that patients feel they are becoming part of something that is significant to themselves and to the sustainability of healthcare systems, as detailed earlier.

In the class, our teachers aim to hold an inclusive space, where all are welcome, regardless of gender, age, ethnicity or sexuality. With chair versions of every practice, people less able to move onto the floor and wheelchair users are welcome. The Yoga4Health programme takes a non-denominational approach and avoids espousing any particular belief system. When spiritual matters are brought into class they are discussed openly and care is taken to not alienate those of any faith or none.

This inclusive approach to teaching is reflected in the posture practices included in the protocol. Every class begins and ends in a chair, with those who are physically able enough moving down to a yoga mat. Chair and mat instructions for the physical practice are given simultaneously. There are also regular reminders that the yoga practice must meet individual needs and that there is no point striving to do an unsuitable practice. Teachers create a non-competitive space in which each student practises appropriately and thereby gets the maximum benefit from the yoga practice. We rely on the skill and sensitivity of our teachers to create this environment every single week of the programme – being there in good time to welcome patients to class, facilitating a healing yoga session, managing discussion skilfully and then closing the session. Chairs and mats are organized into rows, rather than a circle. Some patients attending for reasons linked to stress and anxiety would find it too intense to be organized in a circle, facing other students.

Yoga4Health teachers always ask for consent before touching a patient in class. Some teachers offer hands-on adjustment to help patients experience a yoga posture more effectively, but the patient's right not to be touched is always honoured and consent must always be given first. Some teachers may use Yes Please/No Thanks consent tokens to empower patients to control this consent on a moment-by-moment basis.

THE GATEWAY OF THE PHYSICAL BODY

The Yoga4Health programme is not primarily about physical practice. Yoga postures (*asanas*) are a highly effective way of maintaining full range of motion in joints, stretching tight muscles, releasing tension held in the body and improving posture. On a subtle level, physical release of tension in the muscles and fascia can lead to a feeling of healing, unblocking energy and an improvement in the mind-body connection. Historically, the path of Hatha Yoga (which includes all the posture practice we see today) was an attempt to purify the physical body and use it to prepare for the higher practices of meditation where the mind could be worked on directly.

In the Yoga4Health protocol, we do not teach strong physical practice and instead aim to create mindful breath-led movement that will draw the patient into a deeper connection with their felt experience and be an effective way of quietening and focusing their minds.

Every physical practice included in the protocol is there for a reason. Its creation involved comprehensive discussion and a process of sifting – rather like panning for gold – in which only the best nuggets of effective yoga practice were chosen. The result is that every significant joint in the body is mobilized and invited to move through its pain-free range of motion for joint health. Major muscles are stretched, and significant muscles for spinal and core support strengthened. All traditional yoga movements are included: forward bends, backward bends, side bends, twists, balances and mild inversions.

At the end of each session, we want the patients to feel that their physical body is in a state of balance and ease, or as close to that as possible.

The Yoga4Health protocol involves a great deal of progression through the ten weeks in terms of theme, breathing practices and relaxation. However, the physical practice remains by and large the same every week. This provides an anchor and enables patients to become familiar with the sequence of postures quickly, so that they can think more about their breath and the theme for that week's class.

However, there is some leeway for progression within the physical practice. For example, patients start with a simple one-breath balance in Week 1 and progress, if able, to more challenging balances in later weeks. In early weeks of the course when the Yoga4Health teacher spends more time demonstrating unfamiliar practices, there may not be time to teach the entire physical protocol. So more of the protocol can be included as the course goes on.

We also emphasize to our teachers that the physical practices in the protocol should be taught as sensitively as possible to meet the needs of the patients in their group. The same chair or mat practices are taught on all courses for the purposes of standardization. Modified versions (more gentle versions) of particular practices may be taught.

This ensures that the posture practice is a gateway to a new way of being and not an end in itself.

HOW PATIENTS JOIN YOGA4HEALTH PROGRAMMES

Part of the training to become a Yoga4Health teacher involves understanding social prescribing and taking on the role of a yoga social-prescribing champion in their local community. The way in which social prescribing is organized varies widely. In some areas, it is well-developed; in others, less so.

Discovering the key players in your own social-prescribing scene and forming a network of connections for collaborative working is an important part of the role. This work can be time consuming and involve a lot of unpaid effort. However, our teachers are dedicated to helping others, and they have found it enriching to meet like-minded people in their community working in different areas of social prescribing.

There are some simple steps that all our teachers take when trying to set up Yoga4Health Yoga on Prescription programmes.

- Making contact with Social Prescribing Link Workers.

- Making contact with GP practice managers and any GPs with an interest in yoga; having an advocate on the inside is helpful.

- Connecting to Patient Participation Groups, and giving talks to them and other community groups such as the Women's Institute (WI), University of the Third Age (U3A) and others to get known in the local community.

- Writing articles for the local press or local magazines about Yoga4Health.

- Offering free taster sessions to local NHS staff, Link Workers and patients, for example around National Self Care Week.

- Contacting the local authority team responsible for promoting physical activity and health in the area. This can be a source of grant funding to support Yoga4Health programmes.

- Connecting to any Community Interest Companies (CICs) that might be delivering social-prescribing programmes locally.

- Placing Yoga4Health leaflets in healthcare settings and suitable public places such as the community library.

Whatever links are made, the most crucial ones are with the PCNs in England and Wales and with Health Boards and GP practices in Scotland. PCNs are based on one or more GP practices covering 30,000–50,000 patients, together with pharmacies, social care and mental health services to create a more joined-up service. Yoga4Health is a GP/Link Worker referral programme, and its strength comes from working in partnership with the local NHS. Patients can self-refer onto the programme, but many of these first hear about Yoga4Health via their family doctor or a surgery visit.

We should be aware that Yoga4Health – like other social-prescribing projects – is not directly connected to the NHS. No patient records are passed from the NHS to Yoga4Health teachers, and all data gathering is done completely separately, anonymously and in line with GDPR (UK) Data Protection Regulations. This means that all health information necessary to teach the referred patients safely is gathered by the Yoga4Health teacher themselves. The only external sharing of data is with the patient's family doctor so that their participation on the programme can be added to their patient notes. This will become important if the NHS wishes to track the impact on patient appointments of social-prescribing activities (as one of the aims is to reduce pressure on healthcare services). The British Medical Association issued guidance to hospitals and GP practices in 2019 that listed the benefits to the NHS of social-prescribing schemes leading to improved self-care among patients.

- Fewer hospital admissions and A&E attendances.

- Fewer outpatient appointments.

- Fewer GP consultations.

- Reduced reliance on medical prescription. (British Medical Association, 2019)

Such benefits can only be measured accurately by informing a patient's GP of their participation on the Yoga4Health programme, and that information being recorded in patient records. We obtain permission to do this and to gather data from each patient on a range of measures, including physical and mental health, and social connection. This data is anonymized and sent to YIHA centrally to support the evidence base. Patients sign a data policy statement that makes clear how their personal data will be used and states clearly that no data is ever passed on to a third party, apart from the notification to their GP.

Once approved to join a Yoga4Health course, the patients arrive on Week 1 for their first experience of practising the Yoga on Prescription protocol. Many of them will not have realized at that point that the main transformation they are about to experience is in their minds.

Yoga4Health Patient Pathway

Patient wishes to participate in the Yoga4Health ten-week programme

Patient completes Self-Referral Form including health/medical information

Patient completes Referral Form with GP or Link Worker

Patient completes Yoga4Health Medical Form

Patient is interviewed over phone by Yoga4Health teacher to discuss suitability and practical matters regarding participation in the ten-week programme

Induction, including data protection and Yoga4Health Patient Benchmark Data Form (on or before Week 1)

Ten weeks of classes. Patient completes Yoga4Health Patient Evaluation Form (after Week 9 or at Week 10 session)

Yoga4Health teacher collates Benchmark Data Forms into anonymized summary to build the evidence base for Yoga4Health

REFERENCES

Bandura, A. (1997). *Self Efficacy: The Exercise of Control.* New York: Worth.

British Medical Association (2019). *Social Prescribing: Making it Work for GPs and Patients.* Accessed on 9/9/2021 at: www.bma.org.uk/media/1496/bma-social-prescribing-guidance-2019.pdf.

Cartwright, T., Richards, R., Edwards, A. and Cheshire, A. (2019). *Yoga4Health on Social Prescription: A Mixed Methods Evaluation.* London: University of Westminster.

Gardner, B. and Rebar, A. (2019). 'Habit formation and behavior change.' *Oxford Research Encyclopedia of Psychology.* Accessed on 9/9/2021 at: https://oxfordre.com/psychology/view/10.1093/acrefore/9780190236557.001.0001/acrefore-9780190236557-e-129.

National Institutes of Health (2017). *Science of Behaviour Change.* Accessed on 9/9/2021 at: https://commonfund.nih.gov/behaviorchange.

NHS England (2021). *Module 1: PAM.* Accessed on 9/9/2021 at: www.england.nhs.uk/wp-content/uploads/2018/04/patient-activation-measure-quick-guide.pdf.

Science of Behaviour Change (2021). *The Method.* Accessed on 9/9/2021 at: https://scienceofbehaviorchange.org/method.

Streeter, C. C., Gerbarg, P. L., Brown, R. P., Scott, T. M., *et al.* (2020). 'Thalamic gamma aminobutyric acid level changes in major depressive disorder after a 12-week Iyengar yoga and coherent breathing intervention.' *Journal of Alternative and Complementary Medicine 26,* 3, 190–197.

University of Rochester Medical Center (2021). *Journaling for Mental Health.* Accessed on 9/9/2021 at: www.urmc.rochester.edu/encyclopedia/content.aspx?ContentID=4552&ContentTypeID=1.

CHAPTER 3

Changing Your Mind

If you can change your mind, you can change your life.

William James, American psychologist and philosopher (1842–1910)

YIHA takes an evidence-based approach to yoga. However, this does not sever the connection to the yoga tradition. Indeed, we would argue that yoga's representation in modern society is strengthened by the underpinning of research and evidence. Advocating for a holistic model for health brings together the insights of Eastern spiritual practice and teachings and Western medicine, to the benefit of both.

We see interest in bringing a scientific perspective to leaders in yogic and Buddhist traditions. His Holiness the Dalai Lama, Tenzin Gyatso, the 14th Dalai Lama, is a strong proponent of the interface between science and meditation. In 2004 he collaborated with Richard Davidson and Francisco Varela, founding the Mind and Life Institute. The organization contributed to the emerging belief that mind-body practices could offer great value in the modern age and that through scientific inquiry we can better understand their applications and lend credibility to their value for individuals and healthcare systems alike (Mind and Life Institute, 2021). Mind and Life Institute conferences in Dharamsala in India have helped to build a bridge between science and spiritual practice. Similarly, attention to science is seen in the yoga community, where leaders Sri Sri Ravi Shankar supports regular scientific investigation of his *Sudarshan Kriya*, while Nagendra founded the Swami Vivekananda Yoga Anusandhana Samsthana, a yoga-therapy institute that conducts research into the efficacy of yoga.

At YIHA, we hold similar views about the symbiotic relationship between yoga and science and seek to match the core teaching of the tradition with modern perspective language, and an appreciation of psychophysiology.

THE YOGA TRADITION

The whole of yoga rests on the foundation of Patanjali's 2000-year-old teaching that we can only truly know ourselves and find peace when we control the activity of the mind and bring it into a balanced state of steadiness. Practical techniques are offered to achieve this aim. Then – according to Patanjali – we can experience an unchanging centre of stillness, or pure consciousness, undisturbed by interrupting thoughts (which Patanjali calls the "*vrittis*"). This approach is based on a philosophical paradigm which postulates that our "true Self" lies beneath our thoughts and is unchanging *purusha* (see below).

In an age in which depression, anxiety and stress are rife, we are beginning to appreciate how vital mental training is. We know that evoking mental relaxation is vital to our wellbeing. Scattered and proliferating or ruminative thoughts take us away from the present moment – and often off into anxieties, where we are lost in fears about the future or painful reminders of the past as found in depressive mood. Steadying the mind and exerting a measure of control over the flow of thoughts that arise is a fundamental skill of yoga, and it leads to greater wellbeing. These techniques are also found in the mindfulness tradition, in which a copious body of research reveals the value of cultivating the mind and present-moment awareness. The working definition of mindfulness in healthcare, put forth by Jon Kabat-Zinn, is "paying attention, on purpose, in the present moment, non-judgmentally" (Oxford Mindfulness Centre, n.d.). Yoga practice and mindfulness naturally overlap, so we can extrapolate some findings from mindfulness to what happens within the practice of yoga.

A review of 136 randomized control trials on mindfulness training for improved mental health and wellbeing found that mindfulness techniques worked for most people in most settings (University of Cambridge, 2021). In a report published in the journal *PLOS Medicine*, researchers from the Department of Psychiatry at the University of Cambridge found that in most community settings, compared with doing nothing, mindfulness reduced anxiety, depression and stress, and increased feelings of wellbeing (Gotink *et al.*, 2015). According to the American Psychological Association, mindfulness reduces rumination, stress and emotional reactivity, boosts working memory and improves focus, cognitive flexibility and relationship satisfaction.

MAKING YOGA PHILOSOPHY RELEVANT

People who are new to yoga may be worried that they will experience teachings wrapped up in (what they would see as) spiritual ideas that seem too far-fetched. They may be reassured to discover that yoga is based on one of the six classical schools of Indian philosophy. Samkhya is an ancient approach to reality that is largely rationalist and makes little mention of God (however, the concept of *Ishwara* – supreme being – is mentioned). Instead, Samkhya states that the only reliable means of gaining knowledge is through perception, inference and the testimony of reliable sources. This is one reason why yoga is sometimes described as a science of the body-mind.

In the Samkhyan view of the universe, everything is either *purusha* (pure consciousness) or part of an elaborate taxonomy of *prakriti* (matter). This dualist view of the world suggests that a living person is an example of *purusha* having become bonded to *prakriti* – in this case a physical body – through the process of incarnation. The bonding to *prakriti* gives rise to Ego and a stream of thoughts in the mind generated by sensory input. A multitude of thoughts has the effect of hiding our true nature under veils of false reality, or delusion. We are literally lost in our thoughts.

We may identify as a parent, an engineer or a yoga teacher. We say that we are this or that, but yoga and Samkhya declare that these are superficial labels, used to present ourselves to the world. The ultimate aim of life, according to Samkhya, is to know that you are the unchanging *purusha* of pure consciousness, described in other yogic texts as *ananda*, or bliss.

Patients, along with almost everyone else, will not wish to abandon their carefully constructed identities, and family lives, to head off to a remote cave to meditate on the essential nature of their being! However, they may benefit from moving beyond an entrenched identity and instead creating a new sense of self that feels more peaceful and open.

That transition is likely to include experiencing increased clarity that arises from a less cluttered mind. In moments of heightened mindfulness in postures, breathing practices and relaxation, patients may experience a profound stillness that transcends the busy mind and helps them feel more resilient, grounded and present. This stillness is often a primary reason for practising yoga (once experienced) and has been cited since time immemorial.

This sense of being grounded in the essence of ourselves is the quiet clear mind that embodies the state of yoga (union) described by Patanjali and written about in the Samkhya texts. It is reconnection with a fundamental truth – according to yoga – that we are not our thoughts, nor are we defined by our thoughts. Instead, we are something deeper and unchanging, and through practice, this knowledge arises naturally.

We mentioned, in the introduction, the eight limbs of yoga set out by Patanjali in his Samkhya-inspired treatise on yoga. The last four internal limbs are:

- *pratyahara* – withdrawal of the senses

- *dharana* – concentration

- *dhyana* – meditation

- *samadhi* – superconscious state.

People may not associate a modern yoga class with these qualities. However, if we think about what takes place, we see that it is an experience that correlates very closely with three of these final four limbs. In yoga, we contain our senses (*pratyahara*) by minimizing external inputs through the eyes and ears by listening only for the instructions of the teacher in a quiet and peaceful setting. By focusing on what we experience in the yoga postures and on maintaining a steady breath and a steady gaze (*drishti*), we hone our skills of concentration (*dharana*). These two steps give us the experience of a steadier mind that is completely absorbed in the present moment, which in turn prepares us to lie down and experience a deep relaxation or to sit in meditation (*dhyana*). We may not expect our patients (and probably not ourselves) to enter the final stage of a superconscious state, but they may have the sense of connection and a greater feeling of oneness concomitant with *samadhi*.

In a Yoga4Health class, patients are likely to have a range of experiences, from simple concentration to more settled states of mind that we might describe as meditative. Whatever state of mind is achieved, all patients go through a process of experiencing practices designed to help them steady their minds and learn how to manage the overwhelmed and reactive mind. Through off-the-mat skills offered in each class, and guidance on home practice, they are encouraged to recreate this positive mental state at any time in their daily lives by using their yoga toolkit.

Patients may believe they are coming to class for one set of reasons, but the most powerful transformation they are likely to experience is that of the mind (and, as we saw earlier, relatively new disciplines like psychoneuro-immunology are demonstrating how a person's state of mind directly affects the functioning of their immune system). In a 2020 survey of primary reasons people attend a yoga class, physical fitness was high on the list (Cartwright *et al.*, 2020). However, as time goes by, motivations change. Many patients begin to say they come to reduce stress and anxiety, and connect to the spiritual aspects of life (*ibid.*). However, long-held patterns of thinking – so-called "mind habits" – take considerable effort to overcome and rewire. That is why we place so much emphasis on the importance of a daily home practice.

Patanjali's *Yoga Sutras* also declare that progress can only be made with sustained practice over a considerable period of time. That is what we aim to achieve with the patients on our programmes – through ongoing resource access and signposting to a suitable local class when their ten-week programme ends.

NEUROPLASTICITY

In 1948, the Polish neuroscientist Jerzy Konorski coined the term "neuroplasticity" to describe the changes he observed in the structure of neurons. His work built on much older research. As long ago as 1793, the Italian anatomist Michele Vincenzo Malacarne demonstrated by dissection that training one individual from a pair of animals led to structural changes in the cerebellum. In 1890, William James was writing in *The Principles of Psychology* that the brain of adults exhibited "plasticity" (James, 2013). Santiago Ramón y Cajal (1852–1934) earned the nickname "the father of neuroscience" after winning the Nobel Prize in 1906 for his work on discrete cells of the nervous system, and he became interested in neuroplasticity. This is particularly ironic as he strongly held that the adult brain could not change and was tragically limited by a preordained structure developed in childhood. However, he also published a seminal text expressing the nonpathological changes that occur in the structure of adult brains (Fuchs and Flügge, 2014). He told the Royal Society in London in 1894 that "the ability of neurons to grow in an adult and their power to create new connections can explain learning". In two strokes, Ramón y Cajal both set science back and launched it forward!

It was only in the 1960s, following work on rats and later monkeys, that Marian Diamond demonstrated that the adult brain could change. Modern findings tell us that neurological change can occur in each moment. Even as you read this book and gather new facts and ideas, microscopic neural connections are being made. The brain is in a state of constant dynamic change. These neuroplastic changes happen in a few different ways: neurons within the brain can grow new connections to neurons they did not previously communicate with, allowing for new thoughts, behaviours or capacities; neurons can increase their connections with each other, more deeply embedding tendencies, or reduce connections, undoing former habits. The capacity of the brain to more deeply embed connections is most famously expressed by Canadian psychologist Donald O. Hebb, who coined the phrase "neurons that fire together wire together" (Hebb, 1949). Finally, and miraculously, certain parts of the brain can birth completely new neurons. This process is known as neurogenesis.

The senior Professor of Neuroscience at Texas A&M University and author of 20 books, Dr William R. Klemm, has described the microscopic anatomical changes in brain structure that take place as we store new learning experiences. Electron microscope images show synaptic growth in the brain, with "dendrite spines" forming on existing dendrites to store new information and becoming activated when the new learning is accessed. Dr Klemm describes this inbuilt system of synaptic development as the way the "brain programmes itself for future capabilities" following learning (Klemm, 2014). Dendrites are tentacle-like structures replete with receptor sites that connect to a whopping 10,000 other potential neurons and receive signals that are then transmitted to the next neuron in the chain of command.

Neuroscience has developed rapidly in the past 70 years. In 1950

Eugene Roberts and J. Awarpara separately identified GABA in the brain, the primary inhibitory neurotransmitter, which amongst many other things helps to inhibit fear-based pathways. This knowledge eventually led to a new class of drugs called benzodiazepines, the most famous of which is Valium. In 1969, the Society for Neuroscience was established in Washington, and by 2021 it boasted a membership of 36,000 across 95 countries. In the 1970s and 1980s, there were a slew of Nobel Prizes for scientists extending the frontiers of our understanding of the brain. In 1970, Julius Axelrod, Bernard Katz and Ulf Svante von Euler shared the prize for their work on neurotransmitters. In 1981, Roger Wolcott Sperry won the Nobel Prize for his work on the functions of brain hemispheres; and in 1994, it was Alfred G. Gilman and Martin Rodbell who scooped the award for their discovery of G-protein coupled receptors and their role in signal transduction across cell membranes. The process of synaptic transmission via chemical messengers was discovered by the Nobel Prize-winning neuroscientist Dr Thomas Südhof.

Neuroscience provides the conceptual framework to explain how complex everyday activities, such as driving a car, can become automatic. When we learn a new skill and use the newly created neural pathways regularly, their firing becomes so efficient and smooth that we do not need to think when undertaking a task. Previously meticulous attention to driving that took all our concentration is replaced by being able to chat or think about other things while still driving a car safely.

By contrast, subjects we studied years ago at school may become a dim memory, with limited knowledge remaining accessible to us. Those neural pathways have been used so infrequently that they have degraded or disappeared altogether.

The plasticity of the brain can be useful in the case of brain injury. A stroke victim may suffer paralysis from damage to a part of the brain that controlled the area of the body affected. However, a course of physiotherapy can be effective at recruiting other (often adjacent) areas of the brain to take over the functions provided by the now non-functioning brain tissue that has been destroyed by the stroke. Norman Doidge's book *The Brain that Changes Itself: Stories of Personal Triumph from the Frontiers of Brain Science* (2007) details many of these cases of remarkable neuroplasticity, including people managing to live their lives despite severe brain trauma or even having a whole hemisphere of the brain missing.

The practice of yoga supports neuroplasticity via a preponderance of mechanisms that foster pronounced change (Madhur Tolahunase, 2018). We know this from different research studies that reveal how the brains of yogis change over time with specific increases in volume in parts of the brain like the hippocampus (Rao, Varambally and Gangadhar, 2013). Research has also demonstrated that one of the biochemicals vital in neuroplasticity, brain-derived-neurotrophic-factor (BDNF), known as the fertilizer of neuroplasticity and neurogenesis, increases with the practice of yoga (Thirthalli *et al.*, 2013). One of the primary factors supporting brain change is new experience, which is often provided by yoga. The more parts of the brain that are recruited, the more pronounced the change. A practice like yoga that involves moving, breathing and mindfulness all together sets the stage for significant neuroplastic changes. The confluence of various postures that are often new for people also recruits a significant amount of neurological real estate, as they require motor activation, motor planning and spatial planning. This means that yoga may actually promote greater neuroplasticity than other activities; only time and lots of research will tell.

During the ten-week Yoga4Health programme, patients learn new skills that co-arise with neurological change. Through continuous practice, these have the potential to be enduring, with deeply connected new neural circuits. In "New neural activity patterns emerge with long-term learning", published in the *Proceedings of the National Academy of Sciences* in 2019, scientists explored the necessary condition for long-term change and how this might influence other faculties (Oby *et al.*, 2019). A collaboration between the University of Pittsburgh and the Carnegie Mellon University, the researchers discovered that new neural activity patterns emerge with long-term learning – in other words, through repetition. It also established a causal link between the new patterns and new behavioural abilities. So, as we teach patients to see things through new vistas, they may also begin seamlessly to change their behaviours.

Based on these findings and many others, if patients wish to change their behaviours, they must maintain their yoga practice. Microscopic connections formed during new learning in adult life that are not based on profoundly intense states (in which deeply embedded pathways are laid down, possibly permanently) will only remain if used regularly.

Some patients also wish to leave behind negative internal dialogues about themselves. The writer and psychologist Dr Deann Ware speaks about the professional challenge of dealing with clients who have had years of negative thoughts looping around their minds, creating stronger and stronger neural pathways that have a detrimental effect and an enduring hold. Many talking therapies seek to address these negative inner dialogues through a process of repeated analysis and personal reflection, engendering new thoughts and behaviours over time. These changes are contingent on the ability of these new perceptions to alter brain functioning.

THE NATURAL CHEMICAL HIGH
OF EMOTIONAL CHANGE

The body is constantly in a state of dynamic flux, and emotions are no exception. Most people have had the experience of how emotions can change in an instant – from calm to rage, from happiness to irritation. A quality that yoga practitioners seek to cultivate is the ability to steady their emotional responses. This can be described as stepping off the emotional roller coaster. Understanding the biochemistry of how waves of emotions sweep through the body will help us to understand why yoga is so effective at promoting emotional regulation and emotional intelligence.

Candace B. Pert contributed a milestone discovery in neuroscience. In 1973, she was a young PhD student working under the guidance of her mentor, Dr Solomon Snyder, on a test-tube experiment to prove the existence of receptors on the surface of human cells. For hundreds of years, people have been taking opiate drugs, like morphine and heroin, for pain relief or to achieve a different state of consciousness. Dr Pert and Dr Snyder hypothesized that these opiate drugs must have an effect because their chemical structure allowed them to latch on to cell receptors in the body and enter the cell. They were right.

Once Dr Pert and Dr Snyder had proved that a chemical "key" fitted a receptor "lock" on the surface of cells to open a pathway into the cell, a new question arose: why did these opiate cell receptors exist? A person taking opiate drugs was taking advantage of these ready-made cell receptors. That meant the body must produce its own natural opiate. The race was on to find the body's own naturally occurring chemical "high".

Endorphins (meaning endogenous morphine) were discovered a year later in 1974 by two groups of scientists. These neuropeptides are produced and stored in the pituitary gland. They inhibit pain signals in the body and contribute to feelings of euphoria. The body's own naturally occurring chemical messenger of happiness, exercise, including yoga practice, triggers the release of endorphins. This is one likely reason why people feel good after doing yoga.

The pioneering work of Dr Pert led to a new understanding about how emotions cascade through the whole body all the time via billions of chemical messengers (which Dr Pert called, in her 1999 book of the same name, the "Molecules of Emotion"). They in turn lock on to billions of cell receptors. These informational molecules provide a mechanism linking every cell in the body and allowing all cells and the brain to communicate through a "psychosomatic network".

It has previously been suggested that consciousness is limited to the brain. However, now that we know that thoughts, feelings and emotions lead to cascades of chemical messengers reaching every part of the body, Dr Pert (n.d.) and others have argued that a holistic view of consciousness involves the whole body. Mind-body therapies, such as yoga, appear to work very effectively because they make use of this whole-body perspective. Your state of mind affects the whole of your body, and the state of your body affects the mind.

GABA

GABA is the brain's primary inhibitory neurotransmitter. A complex chemical that can influence various pathways, GABA is best known for inhibiting fear-based pathways. Low levels of GABA have been linked to anxiety, depression, PTSD, epilepsy and chronic pain.

A study published in the *Journal of Alternative and Complementary Medicine* in March 2020 (building on earlier studies from 2007 and 2010) found that in a depressed patient population, practising Iyengar Yoga and Coherent Breathing® could increase levels of GABA in the short term (Streeter *et al.*, 2020). One class per week helped to maintain elevated GABA levels in the brain; however, practising twice a week led to a significant additional spike and more profound reductions in depression (*ibid.*). Coherent Breathing is taught during Weeks 8, 9 and 10 in the Yoga4Health programme.

Notably, once Streeter found that yoga increased GABA at statistically significant levels, she conducted a follow-up study that found yoga increased GABA more than a walking group in the same university gym, where both exercises were metabolically matched (Streeter *et al.*, 2010). This important second study indicated that yoga offered neurological benefits above and beyond other forms of movement practice.

Drawing on her 2007 and 2010 research on GABA, Streeter teamed up with long-time friend and colleague Dr Patricia Gerbarg to better understand how yoga might increase GABA and the possible enduring effects. Both practising psychiatrists were intrigued by how patients might receive life-changing experiences and perceptions over a short period of intense yoga practice. Together, they developed a hypothetical model, which now rings true when read through the vista of new findings. Via the practice of yoga, a specific nerve, the vagus (to be discussed further in the next chapter), receives signals from the body, and lungs in particular. These stimulate an entry point in the base of the brain, the medulla oblongata. This input triggers a large release of GABA. In certain brain structures, this GABA reduces, via inhibition, fear and fear reactivity. In other structures associated with the ability to perceive reality in new ways, the prefrontal cortex, and the part of the brain associated with our felt perception of self, the insula, GABA inhibits old patterns, allowing for innovative thought and feeling. This may be why we emerge from a yoga class and see things from new angles while also feeling relaxed as the GABA pulses through the brain. However, this moment of epiphany can wear off as we return to the networks that signal fear, anxiety, worry and old thoughts.

This is where the second aspect of their hypothesis becomes all the more important. When we repeatedly increase release of GABA, through daily yoga practice, this chemical actually alters neurological pathways, leading to more permanent changes in self and other constructs as it alters pathways in the brain. Over time, we feel differently and think differently. Certainly, the yogis of old professed that their practice led to the very changes Dr Streeter and Dr Gerbarg describe.

CHANGING MINDS ON THE
TEN-WEEK PROGRAMME

All aspects of the Yoga4Health programme are likely to have an impact on the minds of patients: the weekly classes and home practice; postures; breathing; relaxation; social connection. However, the impact of the programme is increased by the interweaving of ten different cumulative themes and psycho-educations that are taught on the ten-week programme to support positive change. This is the part of the programme that works directly on the mind.

- Week 1 – Body and breath awareness – noticing where we feel our breath in our bodies, how it affects how we feel and becoming acquainted with it. Connecting mind and body to honour individual needs.

- Week 2 – Grounding – feeling the touch of the body on the ground. Exploring the idea of connection to the earth and stability and steadiness in our body, breath and mind.

- Week 3 – Grounding – inhaling up from the ground, exhaling back down to the ground. Using the tool of a long exhale to enhance feelings of connection to the ground, while activating the vagus nerve to reduce heart rate.

- Week 4 – Grounding – inhaling ocean breath up from the ground and exhaling long ocean breath back down to the ground. Continuing to explore and develop feelings of embodiment, foundation and connection to the earth, while benefiting from the vast positive effects of ocean breath.

- Week 5 – Spaciousness – inhaling, exhaling, pause/space. Exploring the space at the end of the exhale, which may be a moment when a greater sense of stillness is experienced.

- Week 6 – Spaciousness – noticing the position of the shoulders and rolling them back and down. Using inhale, exhale, pause to find space in the shoulders in every part of the class. Feelings of space in the body and breath, which leads to the experience of space in the mind.

- Week 7 – Awareness of bodily sensations – refining our understanding of what we feel in our bodies to support more effective self-care. Knowing when we are hungry and when we are full. Becoming more able to meet our needs to be healthy and happy.

- Week 8 – Balance – focusing on the breath. Breathing with the chimes, using the 6:6 rhythm of Coherent Breathing with a chime or piano track to support relaxation, resilience and, most importantly, heart rate variability (HRV). HRV is a vital measure of mental health, cardiovascular health and even social connectedness, so it is uniquely important to the groups we work with.

- Week 9 – Change – noticing the beginning and end of inhalation and exhalation. Noticing how breath, sensation and thoughts arise and fall away. Sensation, thoughts and feelings are not permanent. Everything can change in this moment and in our lives. Coherent Breathing is threaded through.

- Week 10 – Connection – we are all breathing together; we are all connected by breath. Appreciating connection to ourselves through yoga practice, and social connection – to others in the group, our families, communities and the planet. Yoga means union, means connection. Coherent Breathing is threaded through.

Our Yoga4Health teachers take five minutes at the start of each class to introduce these weekly themes, which are then threaded through every part of the class that follows. Coherent Breathing is practised throughout.

As we have seen, the themes link closely to the breath – and the breath is at the centre of all yoga practice.

REFERENCES

Cartwright, T., Mason, H., Porter, A. and Pilkington, K. (2020). 'Yoga practice in the UK: A cross-sectional survey of motivation, health benefits and behaviours.' *BMJ Open*, 10.1136.

Doidge, N. (2007). *The Brain that Changes Itself: Stories of Personal Triumph from the Frontiers of Brain Science*. London: Penguin.

Fuchs, E. and Flügge, G. (2014). 'Adult neuroplasticity: More than 40 years of research.' *Neural Plasticity*, 541870.

Gotink, R. A., Chu, P., Busschbach, J. J., Benson, H., Fricchione, G. L. and Hunink, M. G. (2015). 'Standardised mindfulness-based interventions in healthcare: An overview of systematic reviews and meta-analyses of RCTs.' *PloS One 10*, 4, e0124344.

Hebb, D. O. (1949). *The Organisation of Behaviour.* New York: Wiley.

James, W. (2013). *The Principles of Psychology.* New York: Cosimo Classics. First published 1890.

Klemm, W. R. (2014). *Mental Biology: The New Science of How the Brain and Mind Relate.* New York: Prometheus.

Madhur Tolahunase, R. S. (2018). 'Yoga- and meditation-based lifestyle intervention increases neuroplasticity and reduces severity of major depressive disorder: A randomized controlled trial.' *Restorative Neurology and Neuroscience*, 1–20.

Mind and Life Institute (2021). *Insights.* Accessed on 8/9/2021 at: www.mindandlife.org/insights.

Oby, E. R., Golub, M. D., Hennig, J. A., Degenhart, A. D., *et al.* (2019). 'New neural activity patterns emerge with long-term learning.' *Proceedings of the National Academy of Sciences 116*, 30, 15210-15215. Accessed on 8/9/2021 at: www.pnas.org/content/116/30/15210.

Oxford Mindfulness Centre (n.d.). *Paying Attention: On Purpose, in the Present Moment, with Interest and Care.* Accessed on 15/10/2021 at: www.oxfordmindfulness.org/wp-content/uploads/2020/06/Paying-Attention-Handout-10_06_2020.pdf.

Pert, C. (n.d.). *The Institute for New Medicine.* Accessed on 15/10/2021 at: https://candacepert.com/the-institute-for-new-medicine.

Pert, C. B. (1999). *Molecules of Emotion.* New York: Pocket Books.

Rao, N. P., Varambally, S. and Gangadhar, B. N. (2013). 'Yoga school of thought and psychiatry: Therapeutic potential.' *Indian Journal of Psychiatry 55*, Suppl. 2, S145–S149.

Streeter, C. C., Gerbarg, P. L., Brown, R. P., Scott, T. M., *et al.* (2020). 'Thalamic gamma aminobutyric acid level changes in major depressive disorder after a 12-week Iyengar yoga and coherent breathing intervention.' *Journal of Alternative and Complementary Medicine 26*, 3, 190–197.

Streeter, C. C., Whitfield, T. H., Owen, L., Rein, T., *et al.* (2010). 'Effects of yoga versus walking on mood, anxiety, and brain GABA levels: A randomized controlled MRS study.' *Journal of Alternative and Complementary Medicine 16*, 11, 1145–1152.

Thirthalli, J., Naveen, G. H., Rao, M. G., Varambally, S., Christopher, R. and Gangadhar, B. N. (2013). 'Cortisol and antidepressant effects of yoga.' *Indian Journal of Psychiatry 55*, Suppl. 3, S405–S408.

University of Cambridge (2021). *Mindfulness Can Improve Mental Health and Wellbeing – But Unlikely to Work for Everyone.* Accessed on 8/9/2021 at: www.cam.ac.uk/research/news/mindfulness-can-improve-mental-health-and-wellbeing-but-unlikely-to-work-for-everyone.

CHAPTER 4

How Breath Supports Health and Wellness

The breath is the intelligence of the body.

T. K. V. Desikachar

Renowned yoga teacher T. K. V. Desikachar is among many iconic figures in the yoga tradition to assert that breathwork lies at the heart of yoga. This legacy is seen in the tens of thousands of yoga teachers all over the world who regard the simple act of breathing – carried out between 17,000 and 23,000 times a day – as an essential tool for positive change in our bodies and mind.

Breathing can be deep or shallow, smooth or uneven, rapid or slow. Breath may be consciously controlled or automatic. Our own breathing pattern is affected by physical, mental, social and emotional factors, as well as a complex web of subtle physiological mechanisms. However, let us begin with the anatomical basics of breathing and how air is moved in and out of the body.

THE ANATOMY OF BREATHING

The main purpose of breathing is to bring oxygen from the environment to our cells. The secondary purpose is to exhale waste products like carbon dioxide, thus maintaining homeostasis within the system.

The physical process of breathing is as follows. Air enters the nasal cavity (more on the importance of the nose below). It then passes the larynx (the voice box, which has tiny muscles that can be contracted if desired to control air flow) and the pharynx. Once the air passes these two structures, it heads down the trachea, also known as the windpipe. The trachea then branches into the left and the right lungs and becomes the bronchi. The bronchi then further divide into smaller tubes called bronchioles, which terminate at air sacs called alveoli. Alveoli is where gas exchange occurs.

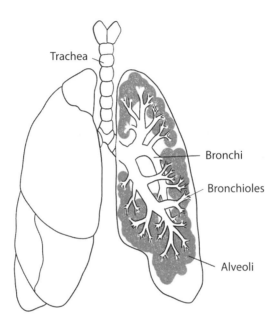

The lungs are impressive, with a surface area the size of a tennis court, and airways within them that if laid end-to-end would stretch from London to Moscow. The key structure in the lungs is the alveoli (we have around 300 million of them!). These alveoli, a collection of the singular alveolus, are often likened to tiny bunches of grapes. Each alveolus is surrounded by capillaries where gas exchange occurs. The capillaries have very thin walls, one cell thick, that allow movement of oxygen and carbon dioxide.

Alveoli contain elastin and collagen, which gives them a spongy and springy quality. This helps to maintain their form and give them elastic recoil to expand on the inhale and recoil on the exhale. A gentle increase in pressure on the lungs, for example from *ujjayi* breathing, further expands an alveolus, supporting gas exchange.

The lungs are divided into lobes. The right lung has three lobes, while the left lung has only two. The smallest branch of the bronchial airways, the bronchioles, are surrounded by smooth muscle and therefore have the capacity to dilate or contract. Contracted bronchioles will partially obstruct the flow of air in and out of the lungs, as seen in people with asthma.

Although breathing is a continuous process, let us imagine that respiration starts with an inhale. Inhalation is initiated by nuclei in the brainstem as they monitor levels of carbon dioxide and oxygen, determining when we need to rid the body of carbon dioxide and refuel it with oxygen. A signal is then sent from the brain via the phrenic nerve to the main muscle of respiration, the diaphragm, initiating contraction. The vagus, the major parasympathetic nerve, also innervates the diaphragm, sending and receiving signals, but it is not directly involved in movement.

The downward movement of the diaphragm results in a negative pressure gradient in the lungs as compared with the external environment (basically, because the lungs now have a lot more space and this reduces the amount of pressure inside the lungs). The result of this action is that air gets pulled into the lungs via the airway due to the principle of diffusion, where substances naturally travel from an area of higher concentration to one of lower concentration.

We can grasp this process if we think about blowing up a balloon. Inflation increases the pressure inside the balloon. If we release the nozzle, the air rushes out to equalize with the pressure outside – leaving a limp uninflated balloon. Our breathing muscles employ this law of physics by alternately decreasing and then increasing air pressure in the lungs – resulting in air rushing in and out of the body.

When the diaphragm contracts and flattens, there is increased space in the thorax for the inhale. When the diaphragm relaxes and moves upwards, the lungs deflate due to their elastic recoil and the gentle pressure of the diaphragm moving upwards as it returns to its relaxed position.

When the diaphragm moves downwards during inhalation, it pushes on the organs below, causing them to be displaced (distended somewhat). This leads to the appearance of what we call "belly breathing". However, we never actually breathe into the belly, as there are no lungs in the lower belly. The internal organs, notably the digestive tract, enjoy a nice massage during belly breathing. This is one of the benefits that yoga often attributes to diaphragmatic breathing.

When a person breathes without fully utilizing the diaphragm, it may only contract downwards by 2 cm. With full diaphragmatic breathing, this movement may increase to up to 10 cm, giving the diaphragm a nice workout.

Although the diaphragm is the main muscle in the process of breathing, it certainly does not work alone. At rest, in a healthy person, the external intercostals can also assist with inspiration, elevating the ribs upwards and outwards and expanding the thorax. This expansion applies pressure to the lower lung wall, supporting the process of oxygen moving into the bloodstream due to increased pressure on the alveoli.

When more rapid breathing is required to meet metabolic needs – such as playing sport or running – the external and internal intercostals work in tandem, rapidly expanding and contracting the ribcage to move air quickly in and out of the lungs, rather like a pair of bellows.

There are other accessory muscles of breathing, including neck and shoulder muscles, that originate in the skull, cervical spine and shoulder blades. These descend to attach to the sternum, clavicle and ribs. When they contract, they support the upward and outward movement of the ribcage. As some of these muscles attach to the scapula, upper arm and shoulder, the shoulder girdle is stabilized by other muscles, like the rotator cuff, so that they can work efficiently in expanding the chest. This is why we might instinctively lean on something for support (hence stabilizing the shoulder girdle) when we are really out of breath.

Why Use Accessory Muscles?

The body's capacity to engage the accessory muscles is necessary and helpful. It supports rapid breathing, which during exercise and a real fight-or-flight situation is important as it improves oxygenation. In this situation, the rate of blood coursing through the body and arriving at the lung walls is very rapid and is coordinated with rapid breathing. To maximally pick up oxygen, we would want to ventilate (breathe) fast and into the chest so that oxygen can be quickly picked up and pumped urgently to cells in need. Another way to explain this is that during intense exercise or fight-or-flight, our perfusion – the rate of the blood arriving at the lung wall – should be aligned with more rapid ventilation.

However, if we are not exercising intensely, fleeing or fighting, rapid and chesty breathing is a poor strategy for getting optimal oxygen into the body, for the following reasons.

- Perfusion and ventilation (the volume of air moved in and out of the body during inhalation and exhalation) will not be well matched. We aren't pumping blood at an accelerated rate, so breathing rapidly will not allow more efficient pickup of oxygen.

- At rest and in an upright position, blood pools at the lower pulmonary (lung) capillaries due to gravity. This means that the place best suited to pick up oxygen is the lower lungs. In contrast, when exercising, the rapid intense beating of the heart does pump the blood rapidly into the upper pulmonary capillaries at a rate that matches speedier and chestier ventilation.

- The lower lungs have more alveoli than the upper lungs. As oxygen can only pass the pulmonary wall via alveoli, non-chesty breathing will naturally support gas exchange better than breathing in the upper lungs.

- Accessory muscles need a good deal of oxygen to operate, just as all muscles do. So, when we engage in unnecessary accessory breathing, a portion of the oxygen we wish to give to other cells of the body is wasted. The diaphragm also uses oxygen for its energy needs, but comparatively less than accessory muscles.

Accessory breathing is not efficient outside of exercise and fight-or-flight and becomes problematic if it occurs at rest. Using the accessory muscles to do the work of the diaphragm is an inefficient way of breathing. Additionally, the use of accessory breathing indicates to the brain that we either are threatened or need to mobilize energy; it therefore stimulates sympathetic response. Chronic chesty breathing keeps the nervous system in a state of alertness. When this becomes a habit, a vicious cycle can set in, whereby the diaphragm is weakened and inhibited by the work of the accessory muscles, and sympathetic arousal becomes chronic.

A dysfunctional breathing pattern using too many accessory muscles may result in a significant amount of tension around the shoulder girdle and neck, and can cause pain and discomfort, including headaches. This in turn can cause more pain, which further provokes sympathetic drive. Additionally, tight accessory muscles are detrimental to good posture, pulling us into a slouching position that further inspires chesty and inefficient breathing. A slouched posture applies pressure around the sternum (breast bone), which in turn applies stresses on nearby cardio-vascular anatomy. The result will again be increased sympathetic drive.

The Abdominals and Pelvic Floor

We have seen that the exhalation in a healthy individual at rest can be mostly passive, with the diaphragm relaxing upwards, assisted by the lung tissue's natural elastic recoil. We have also seen how the internal inter-costals can help to squeeze out air rapidly. However, we also make use of the abdominal muscles to expel air, for example when we cough, sneeze or sing (and we want our exhale to be as complete as possible – pushing out more air than we would at rest – to keep the lovely sound flowing).

When the abdominals contract, they push the abdominal organs inwards and upwards, helping to raise the diaphragm (post-inspiration). The traditional yoga *kriya* of *kapalabhati*/skull shining breath makes use of this abdominal action. Additionally, the abdominal muscles help to maintain good posture for breathing.

The pelvic floor is not a muscle directly involved in exhalation. However, if we think about the dynamics of the abdominals, it makes sense that these muscles play a role. When the abdominals contract and push the abdominal contents inwards, this pressure can be transferred upwards, as we have described, assisting the diaphragm to float back up to its relaxed position. However, the pressure can also be transferred downwards, bulging out the pelvic floor if it is in a relaxed state. In all of nature's elegant designs, this one is slightly questionable (if you have ever sneezed or coughed and let out a bit of wee, you know what we mean!). This is the pressure (called intra-abdominal pressure) being transferred downwards. Conversely, if we purposely contract the pelvic floor, it works synergistically with the abdominal muscles to support the expiration.

If you sit quietly with a steady breath and really focus on the area of the pelvic floor you can feel the increase in downward pressure on it during inhalation, and the sensation of release or lightness on exhale. In a subtle way, the pelvic diaphragm follows the movements of the breathing diaphragm.

INTERNAL RESPIRATION

We left the anatomy of the lungs at the point where air had reached the alveolus within the tens of millions of alveoli. Oxygen travels within the blood, on red blood cells, coursing through the arteries, and it then enters smaller blood vessels and is released to cells. Red blood cells contain a protein called haemoglobin that has a high affinity for both carbon dioxide and oxygen. Haemoglobin picks up carbon dioxide from cells and brings it back to the lungs to be exhaled and collects oxygen from the lungs to bring to cells.

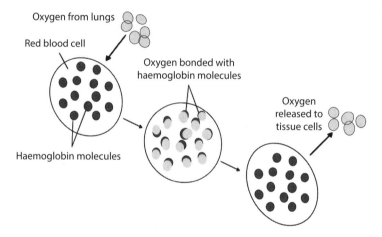

The red blood cells that arrive at the pulmonary walls are part of venous blood from the veins. It has already shared most of its oxygen with cells during arterial flow and is travelling back through the veins to the heart, so it is rich in carbon dioxide. To achieve re-oxygenation, venous blood is pumped into the right atrium of the heart, down the right ventricle and through the pulmonary artery, where it reaches the lungs to drop off carbon dioxide and pick up oxygen. The now oxygen-rich blood is then pumped through the pulmonary vein towards the left atrium, down the left ventricle and back out to the rest of the body, providing life-giving oxygen all over again.

Oxygen Saturation and Breathing

Having a high level of oxygen saturation – saturation of arterial blood (SaO_2) – cited in percentage terms, is important for the healthy functioning of cells. We are mainly concerned with oxygen saturation in arterial blood, as venous blood has already dropped off its oxygen and is returning to the lungs to replenish its reserves. It is generally considered that 94/95–100% saturation is normal and that anything under 92% is problematic. If oxygen saturation dips below 90% in the blood, this is called hypoxemia (below normal blood oxygen) and it can significantly contribute to (or be the result of) ill health. Anything below 80% is so severe it can lead to organ damage.

One of the ways to enhance oxygen levels is to reduce the breathing rate. The average person breathes at a rate of 12–15 breaths a minute (although medical textbooks cite the normative rate at 12–20 breaths per minute). Tidal volume (the amount of air moved in and out of the lungs on each inhale and exhale) is, for the average person, 500 ml. However, when we slow down the rate of breathing, we tend to take more air into the lungs as the slow breath fills the lungs (unless we are actively trying to reduce the intake of air), thereby increasing the tidal volume. Increasing the tidal volume has the following benefits.

- It means that there is slightly more pressure on the alveoli, so their resistance decreases and they open more effectively. In this way, oxygen meets red blood cells more easily.

- The oxygen is pushed into the blood-rich part of the lungs – the base – and can pass through more easily.

- A deeper breath is more efficient. Part of every inhale occupies the conducting airways of the nose, throat and bronchi where there are no alveoli and where no gas exchange can take place; this is known as dead space. Dead space is estimated to be 130–180 ml. When breathing more deeply, we expand beyond the dead space to areas where alveoli are plentiful.

Therefore, by helping a person to reduce their breathing rate, you often help to increase oxygen saturation in those with low or compromised saturation. Dr Luciano Bernardi, a researcher on the forefront of yogic breathing, has demonstrated that slow breathing helps to increase oxygen saturation in many individuals who would otherwise struggle to get oxygen into the blood (Spicuzza *et al.*, 2000). These include individuals:

- climbing at high altitudes

- with chronic obstructive respiratory diseases

- who suffer from heart failure (the heart doesn't pump as it should)

- who suffer from dyspnea (shortness of breath).

Dr Bernardi ascertained that, at rest, the optimal breathing rate for oxygenation is between 5 and 6 breaths a minute (*ibid.*). This magical rate seems to have many far-reaching benefits. Further, he demonstrated that individuals who use this breathing rate are better prepared for vigorous exercise (*ibid.*). Oxygen can get into the system more efficiently. It appears this rate best matches perfusion and ventilation. Long slow inhaling (as we find at this rate) causes a pressure gradient with the descent of the diaphragm that draws venous blood up towards the heart and then to the lungs at a time that the lungs are maximally filled with air. This promotes effective oxygen uptake. In fact, Dr Bernardi has recommended this rate for patients with both cardiovascular and respiratory diseases where a mismatch of perfusion to ventilation is problematic (*ibid.*).

In addition to increasing oxygen levels, slow breathing helps to keep carbon-dioxide levels at a high norm. Although carbon dioxide is often seen as a useless by-product, it is vital for a healthy system. Carbon dioxide helps to dilate blood vessels; hence, it is known as a vasodilator. If levels are too low, it is harder to get oxygen to the brain, as vessels become narrow through vasoconstriction. Notably, when carbon-dioxide levels are higher, haemoglobin releases oxygen more readily to the cells. So, keeping carbon-dioxide levels up is important. When we breathe rapidly or through the mouth, we reduce carbon-dioxide levels, and this may influence oxygen delivery.

On the other hand, the body is vigilant to increases in carbon dioxide, as high levels of carbon dioxide can make the blood acidic and would be dangerous. This is not going to happen due to poor breathing, so do not worry. Nonetheless, the body, and in particular the brain and heart, are very responsive to increases in carbon dioxide and may trigger more rapid exhalations to rid the body of it.

In fact, the body is more receptive to changes in carbon dioxide than to oxygen. However, heightened sensitivity is problematic; remember carbon dioxide plays an important role in the delivery of oxygen to the cells. In many people with respiratory problems like asthma, with mental health issues and with mouth breathing, the nuclei in the brainstem are habitually oversensitive to carbon dioxide, provoking unnecessary and more rapid exhalation. Another way to say this is the mechanism responsible for picking up carbon-dioxide levels and normalizing them, the respiratory chemoreflex, is overactive.

This creates a spiralling issue. Exhaling more rapidly (just quicker than we do in gentle diaphragmatic breathing) is mediated by the SNS. When sympathetic drive is increased, cells synthesize adenosine triphosphate (ATP) faster to meet energy demands. A by-product of this catalytic reaction is carbon dioxide. So greater sympathetic drive means more carbon dioxide. The oversensitive chemoreflex then triggers faster exhalation to rid the body of carbon dioxide, keeping the person in a state of chronic sympathetic drive. At the same time, the ridding of too much carbon dioxide means poor oxygen delivery, and this also causes greater sympathetic activity.

In 2001, Dr Bernardi found that breathing at 6 breaths a minute increased oxygen saturation (for reasons described above) and naturally reduced the sensitivity of the respiratory chemoreflex (Bernardi *et al.*, 2001). This allowed a greater tolerance of carbon dioxide and therefore would be met with greater oxygen delivery. Further, he and various other researchers have discovered that breathing at 5–6 breaths a minute reduces anxiety levels (Schwerdtfeger *et al.*, 2020).

Finally, when done correctly, slow breathing requires little accessory muscle effort, and this may reduce body tension.

RATIO OF INHALE TO EXHALE

We can manipulate the breath to bring about specific effects. For example, we can make the exhale much longer than the inhale, initiating a deep state of calm, or increase the length of the inhale to lift energy. These effects arise, because inhalation and exhalation correspond to the sympathetic and parasympathetic systems, both from a muscular perspective and from a neurophysiological one as well. From a purely muscular perspective the exhalation is passive, unless we are forcing it, and inhalation is active. In addition to this basic phenomenon, the inhale and exhale are linked to the two aspects of the ANS. The ANS has been mentioned previously. It has two branches: the SNS which revs us up; and the PNS which calms us down.

The sympathetic side of the ANS is responsible for the flight or fight response, which evolved to protect humans from danger. When there is a threat, sympathetic nerves can, almost instantaneously, cause changes in the body to prepare us to run away or stand and fight, or freeze. Blood is diverted to muscles, pupils dilate and stress hormones are released.

Unfortunately, modern life can be so intense and overwhelming that many people enter a state of chronic sympathetic response. In this stressed-out state, the whole body works less efficiently, and the immune system is suppressed by stress hormones such as cortisol, epinephrine and norepinephrine. This can lead to fatigue, illness and an elevated risk of chronic diseases, such as cardiovascular disease. Fight-or-flight works well if there is an immediate danger to life – like being chased by a predator – but as a long-term state of being it is damaging to health.

The purpose of the parasympathetic branch of the ANS is to allow us to relax, digest, bond, and build resources for a healthy body and mind. The main mediator of the PNS is the vagus. Vagal activity from the body to the brain can lead to a state of rest and ease. The vagal effects moving from the brain to body are more varied; for example the vagus supports active digestion and sexual arousal.

Every time we exhale the vagus is increasing its signalling to the heart. These signals impede heart rate and the intensity of contraction, so on the exhale the heart rate drops, and the heart gets a brief moment of relaxation. This reduction in heart rate is picked up by the brain, leading to a state of greater parasympathetic activity. On the inhale messaging to the heart via the vagus is slightly reduced and heart rate is increased, as is contraction. If our goal is to relax, as it often is, we want to gently elongate the exhale in relationship to the inhale. Breath has a profound effect on the ANS, which as its name suggests is autonomous, rather than being under direct conscious control.

NOSE BREATHING IS BETTER

We cannot leave the physiology of breathing without looking in more detail at the important role played by the nose, and the pre-eminence of nose breathing in the yoga tradition.

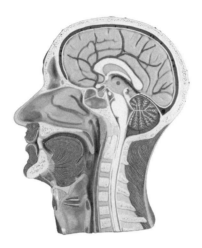

Just inside the nose are the inspiringly named nasal turbinates, also known as nasal concha. These structures are involved in warming, humidifying and filtering the air we breathe. However, their curved seashell-like shape also causes the air we breathe to spin, and any particles, bacteria or other foreign bodies are thrown by the centrifugal force onto the sticky mucus that lines the nose. The delicate nasal lining is just one cell thick, enabling white blood cells to squeeze through into the mucus and devour invaders. Tiny beating cilia in the mucus turn it into a moving carpet, terminating at the back of the nose, where we occasionally swallow. Any remaining would-be invaders are despatched to the stomach to be killed off by the acid there.

The leading Buteyko Breathing teacher Patrick McKeown says:

> Nasal breathing performs at least 30 functions on behalf of the body... Because the nostrils are significantly smaller than the mouth, nose breathing performed while awake creates about 50% more resistance to airflow than mouth breathing. This results in 10–20% greater oxygen uptake in the blood. (McKeown, 2021a, p.104)

The nasal cavity and paranasal sinuses are also where the body produces nitric oxide molecules. The presence of nitric oxide in the breath of humans was not discovered until 1991. It was previously thought to be a harmful toxic gas associated with car exhaust fumes and smog. However, in 1992, *Science Magazine* branded it "molecule of the year". Nitric oxide was shown to be a bronchodilator, meaning that it opens the airways, helping to deliver oxygen to the alveoli.

Nitric oxide also acts as an antiviral, reducing the possibility of pathogens entering the respiratory system. In 1999, two researchers, Lundberg and Weitzberg, reported that nitric oxide inhibits the proliferation of various pathogens in the body, including bacteria and viruses (Lundberg, 1999).

At the seminal Wellness After Covid Symposium in May 2021, several researchers spoke about the supporting role that nasal nitric oxide could play in the battle against Covid-19. Researcher William Bushell and yoga teacher Eddie Stern have collaborated to develop yoga practices that support the resilience and efficient working of the head, nose and respiratory pathways as a way of better defending the body from viruses like Covid-19 that enter the body through the respiratory tract.

Harvesting this naturally created nitric oxide in the body can only take place if we inhale through the nose. For these reasons, it is preferable to breathe through the nose in most circumstances. Incidentally, it has been discovered that humming greatly increases the production of nitric oxide. Perhaps the yogis who developed *brahmari*/bee breath knew more than they were letting on!

Awareness of Breathing

Unless a person times their breathing rate, they may be unaware how often they breathe. A fundamental part of yoga is to create new awareness of breath, with the intention of extending this more mindful habit into everyday life.

Breath control is fundamental to yoga. In an aerobic fitness class, a person will generally be breathing rapidly, without much attention to breathing in a conscious and controlled manner. In other activities, like swimming, there is a much closer alignment of physical movement and breath. In yoga, this is taken a step further. Without the breath, yoga would be an empty practice. The postures would become degraded to physical exercise, and the mind would wander. Yoga is a breath-led practice, and the breath provides a bridge between the body and the mind that allows students to make their journey of transformation.

Breathing in the Yoga Tradition

In asserting the primacy of the breath in the Yoga4Health protocol, we are at one with the yoga tradition. The "life-breath" is repeatedly mentioned in the *Upanishads* – a body of writing dating from the sixth or seventh century BCE and added to for hundreds of years thereafter. In the Upanishadic tradition, breath is also the subtle energy or life force, known as *prana*, which permeates everything and everyone. In other Eastern holistic disciplines, like Tai Chi, this energy is known as *chi* or *ki*.

The traditional view of yoga breathing practices is that their aim is to control and channel this subtle energy, hence the term *pranayama* (*prana* = energy; *ayama* = restrain or control). Patanjali sets out clearly the centrality of the breath:

> Yoga pose is mastered by relaxation of effort, lessening the tendency for restless breathing, and promoting an identification of oneself as living within the infinite breath of life.
>
> From that perfection of yoga posture, duality, such as reacting to praise and criticism, ceases to be a disturbance.
>
> ...In the fourth method of regulating one's breath, prana is extended into the divine life force and the range of prana is felt permeating everywhere, transcending the attention given to either external or internal objects.
>
> As a result of this pranayama, the veil obscuring the radiant supreme light of the Inner Self dissolves. (*Yoga Sutras of Patanjali*, chapter 2, verses 42–47 and 51–52; Stiles, 2021, p.29)

In the Yoga4Health protocol, we invite patients to explore their breath in fine detail; to become intimately familiar with it, including the pauses (or turning points) between inhale and exhale. Often, the biggest change for them is simply connecting to a deeper slower breath and moving from 12–15+ breaths per minute to 5–6 – the rate that is most fruitful in terms of maximally increasing the ventilation-to-perfusion ratio. This radical change in breath tempo has a powerful and positive effect on the body's physiology and supports the relaxation response.

Lung Capacity

One reason why yoga practitioners effectively reduce their breath rate is they learn to access unused lung capacity. This is worth exploring in a little detail, as many people are puzzled or even alarmed at the idea of making such a big reduction in how frequently they breathe. Seeing how efficient slow and low breathing is may be reassuring.

As noted earlier, at rest, the average breath is just 500 ml – or in imperial terms, less than a pint of air. However, an average pair of lungs has the capacity to draw in 4800 ml – more than eight pints. When combined with better posture, slow and low conscious breathing enables students to access this untapped capacity. They learn to stretch their bodies in yoga postures, but also to stretch their breath well beyond its usual length.

The maximum amount of air a healthy adult can breathe in is calculated by taking overall lung capacity of around 6000 ml and subtracting 1200 ml, which is the amount of air that remains in the lungs even after your most thorough exhalation (residual volume). This gives us the figure of 4800 ml of possible air that can enter the lungs. We could define a maximum breath as approximating to around this figure, known as the vital capacity.

Eight-and-a-half pints of air still sounds like lot of air, and it is. The resting rate of 15 breaths per minute of 500 ml of air = 7500 ml of ventilation per minute (minute ventilation). It would take just two maximum breaths of 4800 ml to surpass this rate of ventilation. However, it would be unrealistic (and unhelpful as we shall see) to expect anyone to achieve the high figure of 4800 ml per breath. Nevertheless, even if they were only upping their capacity from 500 ml to a comfortable 1500 ml, it would mean that 5 breaths per minute would lead to the same 7500 ml of ventilation.

IS MORE ALWAYS BETTER?

The "full yogic breath" is still widely taught in yoga-teacher training programmes, based on the premise that the fuller and deeper the breath the better. On YouTube, you can watch the late and great B. K. S. Iyengar demonstrating inhale (which goes on for 48 seconds) and exhale (which lasts for 35 seconds), reinforcing this view.

While there is little doubt that many people would benefit from creating depth, capacity and resilience in their breathing mechanism, there is also compelling evidence that a substantial number of people are chronic over-breathers. The last thing they need is a practice to increase their hyperventilation. Because it is important to recognize over-breathing in yoga students and patients, we are going to explore this further, drawing on insights from the system of Buteyko Breathing. We do not formally teach any Buteyko Breathing techniques on the Yoga4Health protocol, but its theory and method enrich our understanding of breathwork.

Konstantin Buteyko was a Ukrainian doctor who pioneered techniques for people with breathing disorders in the 1950s. He is said to have cured himself of high blood pressure by switching from his long-term habit of deep breathing to reduced breathing.

Professor Buteyko observed that many of his asthma patients were hyperventilating between attacks. He reached the groundbreaking conclusion that the simple act of breathing, so necessary to sustain life, could also be a cause of disease.

The evidence supporting Buteyko Breathing has grown rapidly in recent years, and it is used widely with clients suffering from asthma, anxiety and sleep disorders, including sleep apnea (where the breathing rhythm is repeatedly interrupted during sleep, often accompanied by snoring).

The Buteyko method has benefited from the changing perspective on the role of carbon dioxide in breathing. People enjoyed the benefit of organized bathing in waters rich in carbon dioxide for hundreds of years from the 16th century onwards (it probably also took place much earlier in natural carbon-dioxide hot springs). They bathed to remedy asthma, obesity, anxiety, eczema and other conditions. James Nestor in his book *Breath* says:

> After a brief soak in the thermal waters, bathers would see their skin become rosy and flushed... [Those] with asthma reported a sudden clearness in their breathing. Overweight guests would see flab in their stomach or legs begin to tighten and disappear. (Nestor, 2020, p.174)

After some notable cases where people became ill or died from carbon-dioxide therapies using very high concentrations of the gas, the practice fell out of fashion, and carbon dioxide was dismissed by various authorities as a toxic waste gas.

We explained the fallacy of this view earlier. It is interesting to note that as long ago as 1904, the Danish biochemist Christian Bohr discovered that carbon dioxide facilitates the release of oxygen at a cellular level. He showed that carbon dioxide acted as a catalyst for haemoglobin to release its oxygen payload. When carbon-dioxide levels in the blood are low, the bond between oxygen and haemoglobin strengthens, inhibiting the body from accessing the oxygen it needs. This has become known as the Bohr effect.

People who have a breathing pattern disorder (BPD) that involves over-breathing (defined as breathing in excess of metabolic needs) may have chronically depressed levels of carbon dioxide in their body. This in turn inhibits the ability of their tissues and organs to access the oxygen being carried around the bloodstream. This can be taking place even though they have apparently healthy oxygen saturation levels in the blood leaving their lungs.

According to this approach to breathwork, many people with a long-term BPD have developed a systemic oversensitivity to carbon dioxide (a phenomenon we mentioned earlier that bears repeating). As soon as their carbon-dioxide levels begin to rise – even towards normal range – their body's chemoreceptors are activated to tell them to breathe. This expels more carbon dioxide, perpetuating the problem. Such people may also display outward symptoms of inefficient oxygen transmission at tissue level. These can include coldness in the hands and feet, fatigue, yawning, frequent sighing, coughing, wheezing, nasal congestion, snoring and a feeling of constriction in the airways.

According to the Buteyko method, ascertaining whether someone falls into this category of being a chronic over-breather can be done via a simple test called the "control pause". Following a normal exhale, a person in good health (and not contraindicated for breath holding) will pause their breath and time how long it is before they get a significant urge to breathe in (called "air hunger"). Buteyko teaches that a comfortable breath-hold time after normal exhalation of 25 seconds indicates a functional breathing pattern. In a study of 51 individuals by Professor Kyle Kiesel, those with a comfortable breath-hold time of 25 seconds had an 89% chance that dysfunctional breathing was not present (Kiesel *et al.*, 2017). Asthmatics and those with anxiety conditions frequently present with control pauses of less than 15 seconds. McKeown reports that some patients he has treated with Long Covid can only pause the breath for as little as 5 seconds (McKeown, 2021b).

Buteyko offers a series of practices that support clients to build up their control pause gradually over time and to shift to a habit of reduced breathing, always through the nose. At rest or during light movement, the breath should be silent, slow and low (in the diaphragm) and relaxed. Clients are also recommended to wear mouth tape at night to ensure nose breathing when asleep.

Nowadays, many yoga teachers, complementary therapists and healthcare professionals have trained to become Buteyko Breathing coaches at places like McKeown's Buteyko Clinic International in the Republic of Ireland. The leading International Association of Yoga Therapists member and author of *Restoring Prana*, Robin Rothenberg, is among a growing number of yoga teachers who have integrated the insights of Buteyko into their understanding of yoga breathwork (Rothenberg, 2020).

The Buteyko Breathing approach has highlighted to us the importance of our teachers noticing those patients who enter the programme with an over-breathing habit. We would want to ensure that they practise the long exhale and Coherent Breathing in a way that did not deepen a habit of hyperventilation.

In 2017, there was further evidence to support the view that carbon dioxide plays an important role in physiology when Dr Umesh Pal Singh from the Subharti Medical College in India discovered that the gas also stimulates the vagus nerve and slows heart rate (Singh, 2017).

BREATHING PRACTICES IN THE YOGA4HEALTH PROTOCOL

The posture work taught in each session of the Yoga4Health programme is broadly the same every week, following the sequence set out in the protocol. However, the breathwork develops week by week, with the aim of equipping each student with breathing practices they can use in everyday life as part of their personal yoga toolkit.

It is no surprise that the programme begins with simple breath awareness and cultivating the slow, low and relaxed habit of breathing in and out through the nose that we have seen is so beneficial.

Week 1

During Week 1, patients simply pay attention to their breath. For some of them, this might be the first time in their lives they have done this. It takes them time to gain the habit of slow and smooth conscious controlled breathing – something they will need to practise at home. By noticing the sensations of the breath entering the body, how the body makes space for each inhalation through the action of breathing muscles and the effortlessness of the exhale, a new relationship to breath is established.

During the early weeks of the programme, Yoga4Health teachers are on the lookout for patients with chesty or laboured breathing and may offer individual advice and cues to encourage a shift in breathing patterns.

The first two practices of the protocol – while patients are still sitting in their chairs – aim to cement the relationship to breath. Starting with the palms together in front of the heart, the patients inhale and separate the hands, mirroring the expansion they feel in their bodies of the in-breath. As they exhale, the palms return to their starting position, reflecting the contraction of the exhale. Coordinating breath with movement begins in Week 1 and develops weekly, eventually becoming breath-led movement.

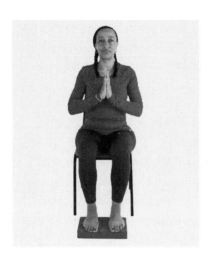 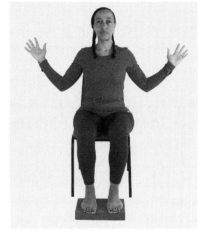

The second physical practice uses a different arm movement to remind students that there are four phases to the breath (something they will be taught explicitly in later weeks). Inhale feels like not only an expansion, but also an upward movement, reflected here in the arms floating upwards. The turning of the palms at the end of the inhale reminds patients that there is a transition between inhale and exhale. The lowering of the arms reflects the departing exhale and the feeling of moving from filling to emptying. Later in the programme, the hand movements will become a place to explore the momentary pauses between inhalation and exhalation, and exhalation and inhalation.

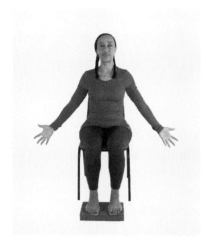 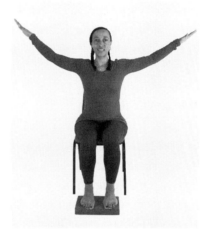

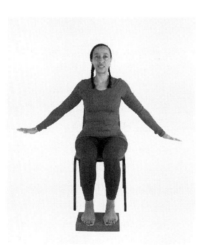

Week 2

In Week 2, the patients begin the first of three weeks of imagining that they are breathing up and down from the ground. This supports the theme of grounding running from Weeks 2 to 4, but also has another purpose. We tend to think about the breath happening within the physical limitations of the lungs. However, by using our imagination, or visualization, we can think about the breath filling the whole of the chest, abdomen, hips, indeed any part of the body. We can also direct breath, in this case up and down from the ground, to give patients an enhanced experience and sensation of embodiment and grounding. The imagination gives the feeling of transcending the physical limitations of breathing, and a deeper expression of breath.

Week 3

In Week 3, we ask patients to begin to learn a more subtle technique of breath control called "ocean breathing". This is our non-Sanskrit description of the yoga *pranayama*, *ujjayi* or victorious breath. It is a familiar and widely used technique in yoga, either as a stand-alone practice or combined with breath and movement.

Ocean breathing is needed in Week 3 because we ask patients to make their exhale longer than their inhale, and this technique supports the lengthened out-breath very effectively. Through this technique, students develop a simple skill to evoke calm, giving them a sense of greater control over their bodies and minds.

Ocean breathing involves a subtle contraction of the laryngeal muscles in the throat where air enters the windpipe in the region of the vocal cords. Almost everyone can do this practice because almost everyone can whisper or sigh, which naturally activates this region. When we sigh the breath out through the mouth with a long controlled "Haaaaa" sound, we are controlling the flow of breath at the throat.

The benefit of exerting this subtle control is that it gives patients an additional tool to slow down the flow of their breath, enabling them to lengthen both the inhale and exhale. Ocean breathing also gets its name from the sound created in the throat by this type of breathing, which can remind people of waves rolling in to shore.

Our teachers deploy a number of strategies to help patients connect to their ocean breath. In Week 3, we begin by only teaching the technique on the exhale. This might be instructed by imagining fogging up a mirror. Another teaching method is to have the group sighing the breath out of the mouth and then asking them to close their mouth halfway through the exhale. Hey presto! The out-breath shifts to the nose, but the sighing sound continues, now more quietly.

It can take some patients a little time to master ocean breathing, so we encourage rather than require it. For some patients with BPDs or coughs, or for whom the practice triggers a negative mental and emotional response, reassurance is given that their usual breath lengthened as best they can is absolutely fine. Breathing in and out of the nose as before, with a slightly longer exhale, is perfectly acceptable. Videos on this breathing technique are made available to patients, and the technique is recapped at the end of Week 3 and the start of other sessions.

Week 4

Week 4 sees the addition of ocean breathing on the inhale as well as the long exhale as patients continue with the theme of grounding. Making sound on an inhale is a little trickier, so again, patients are guided through slow and steady steps to help them experience this sound, often using the mouth as a starting point (sighing the breath in with a "Haaaaa" sound).

Whereas the posture practice remains a relatively fixed anchor week by week, the breathwork develops apace. For students to become familiar and comfortable with these new techniques being learned each week in the early stages of the protocol, home practice is necessary, and strongly encouraged.

Week 5

In Week 5, the theme shifts to spaciousness, but ocean breathing continues, with the addition of a short pause at the end of each exhalation. This is not a breath retention and may only last for a split second for some patients. However, it supports the long exhale by inviting students to carry on breathing out until their exhale has completely died away and then pause...1, 2, for the inhale to naturally arise.

It would not be safe for Yoga4Health patients to explore the sustained breath holding seen in some yoga *pranayamas*, which we would regard as advanced practice. However, patients can experience the same sense of stillness and profound mindfulness that accompanies these short pauses in the breath.

The pauses also help students to define in their minds the phases of the breath and to drop the common habit of clipping the breath. Many people never quite complete their in-breath before they begin to exhale, and do not quite finish their exhale before the next in-breath hurries in. Ocean breath on inhale and exhale slows down the breath. When combined with the pause at the end of the exhale, a truly spacious breath is experienced by patients.

With reference to the benefits of carbon-dioxide tolerance and its importance in breathing mentioned earlier, this slow inhale, exhale, pause is an effective way of bringing about reduced breathing and more likely to support a normalization of carbon-dioxide levels in those who may be carbon-dioxide depleted due to over-breathing. The pause allows a short period in which carbon-dioxide levels are increased in relationship to oxygen and may help with better delivery of oxygen on the next inhale.

At this point, patients are halfway through the ten-week programme and are hopefully beginning to feel major changes in their breath, body and mind as result of the yoga practice and their daily home practice.

Weeks 6 and 7

The same inhale, long exhale, pause with ocean breathing is sustained for Weeks 6 and 7. This technique represents a peak practice in terms of learning to relax, calm down and "let go". By controlling their breath, lengthening the exhale and becoming adept at ocean breathing, patients have learned how to use breath to influence in a positive way the workings of their ANS by triggering the parasympathetic relaxation response.

Weeks 8, 9 and 10

By the time patients arrive for their Week 8 session, they are ready for the final three weeks of breathing practices that mark a change of direction to shift the focus from relaxation to resilience.

However, the vagus nerve is still to the fore. Beneath conscious awareness, the vagus and sympathetic nerves act like a pendulum increasing and decreasing the heart rate (as described earlier, this is known as heart rate variability, HRV). HRV is a vital indicator of physical resilience and psychological resilience. High levels of HRV speak to the strength of both the sympathetic and parasympathetic systems and the ability to flexibly move between the two. Healthy HRV is also concomitant with cardiovascular health and good cognitive control. We can use the influence of breath on heart rate to increase HRV. The effect that breath has on HRV is known as respiratory sinus arrhythmia (RSA).

In Week 8, patients on the Yoga4Health programme learn a new breathing technique that has been shown to be one of the most effective at maximizing HRV.

COHERENT BREATHING
We mentioned Coherent Breathing (or equal breathing) earlier and its physiological benefits. The Coherent Breathing method encourages practitioners to work towards breathing in for 6 seconds and out for 6 seconds, meaning that one breath cycle takes 12 seconds. This leads to a breathing rate of 5 breaths per minute.

However, the breathing is tailored to patient needs, and no strain is put on the breath, so a rate of around 5–6 breaths per minute is recommended in a flexible way. The breath needs to retain a quality of subtlety and flow, and our teachers remain vigilant to support patients whose breath is laboured, chesty or too deep (hyperventilation).

To help patients integrate Coherent Breathing, an audio track of a chime, piano or another sound is played every six seconds during most of the class in Weeks 8–10. This means that the technique is used consistently and not only during the stand-alone breathing practices at the start and end of every session.

The practice is based on the Coherent Breathing technique developed by Stephen Elliott, working with Dee Edmonson (Elliott, 2021).

You can find a wealth of information about the practice at: www.coherentbreathing.com. They have published the books *The New Science of Breath* (Elliott, 2005) and *Coherent Breathing: The Definitive Method* (Elliott, 2008). This technique was further internationally popularized by Dr Brown and Dr Gerberg, authors of *The Healing Power of Breath* and the Breath-Body-Mind system.

Stephen Elliott began researching Coherent Breathing in the 2000s, examining the correlation between breathing, heart rate, electroencephalography and galvanic skin response. He reached the finding that slow, deep, rhythmic breathing facilitated rapid changes in these measures, tending toward parasympathetic response and a meditative state.

Patients on the Yoga4Health programme are taught to practise Coherent Breathing in a step-by-step manner.

Inhale 1, 2

Exhale 1, 2

Inhale 1, 2, 3

Exhale 1, 2, 3

Inhale 1, 2, 3, 4

Exhale 1, 2, 3, 4

Inhale 1, 2, 3, 4, 5

Exhale 1, 2, 3, 4, 5

Inhale 1, 2, 3, 4, 5, 6

Exhale 1, 2, 3, 4, 5, 6

Each count is one second. Once a count of 6 is reached, the soundtrack can be used to cue the breath. However, it is always advised that there is no strain on the breath, so not all patients breathe at the six-second rate.

Practising 5 breaths per minute can be done safely, as there are no retentions. Beginners are encouraged to aim for 3–5 minutes of practice and to increase the length of time from there. Coherent Breathing may also play a role in improving mental health. A study published in March 2017 in *The Journal of Alternative and Complementary Medicine* found that a combination of Iyengar Yoga and Coherent Breathing significantly improved the mood of those suffering major depressive disorders (Streeter *et al.*, 2017). A further analysis of this same study published in 2020 found that this combination also increased levels of GABA (Streeter *et al.*, 2020).

Breathing Practices on the Yoga4Health Ten-Week Programme

Week 1	General breath awareness with a focus on low, slow abdominal breathing.
Week 2	Breathing up and down from the ground.
Week 3	Natural inhalation with elongated exhalation using ocean breath. Breathing up and down from the ground.
Week 4	Inhaling ocean breath, long exhale ocean breath. Breathing up and down from the ground.
Week 5	Inhaling ocean breath, long exhale ocean breath and short pause. Spaciousness in the breath.
Week 6	Inhaling ocean breath, long exhale ocean breath and short pause. Spaciousness in the breath.
Week 7	Inhaling ocean breath, long exhale ocean breath and short pause. Awareness of sensations.
Week 8	Coherent Breathing. Inhaling for 6 seconds and exhaling for 6 seconds. 5 breaths per minute. Balancing the breath.
Week 9	Coherent Breathing. Inhaling for 6 seconds and exhaling for 6 seconds. 5 breaths per minute. Noticing change with each breath.
Week 10	Coherent Breathing. Inhaling for 6 seconds and exhaling for 6 seconds. 5 breaths per minute. Awareness of connection with every breath.

BREATHING, POSTURE AND EMOTIONAL WELLBEING

Yoga teachers and other bodyworkers observe that breath affects posture, and posture affects breath. It is difficult to express your breath fully if your posture is hunched or your shoulders are tight and rolled forwards. Sometimes a rounded back is caused by hereditary factors or spinal problems such as ankylosing spondylitis – arthritis of the spine. However, a sedentary, chair-sitting lifestyle can also be to blame and may be at least partly reversible with yoga.

This rounding may begin with shoulder tightness, which can have a number of causes, including those detailed earlier in the chapter in the "Why Use Accessory Muscles?" section. However, it can also be caused by stress, lack of confidence, trauma and other social and emotional factors that negatively impact mental health. If someone feels threatened by the world, it is no surprise that they might want to curl forwards in their posture and literally hide away the vulnerable front of their body and their heart to protect it. An appropriate non-competitive yoga practice can support people who are addressing underlying social and emotional issues and give them the safe space and awareness to self-care and self-heal through a holistic breath-led practice.

Discovering the breath and gaining control over it – as well as learning techniques that can be used at times of stress – helps students to face life more confidently. This is likely to promote better posture and less tension in the shoulders, and may lead to fewer incidences of lower back pain.

During Yoga4Health classes, the posture of patients is supported using chairs, or yoga blocks if seated on the floor. Good posture, especially a straight spine, will support good breathing, whereas a hunched position may reinforce unhelpful breathing habits.

Most yoga breathing is done sitting up. This reflects the importance given in the yoga tradition to the structure of the physical spine, but also the theory of subtle energy (including *prana*, *chakras*, *nadis* and *kundalini*) that correspond to it. On the Yoga4Health programme, the formal breathing practices are done in an upright position, beginning with everyone on a chair. Each week's breathing technique continues through posture practice, including lying on the floor.

Now it is time to explore the physical practices included in the Yoga4Health protocol.

REFERENCES

Bernardi, L., Sleight, P., Bandinelli, G., Cencetti, S., *et al.* (2001). 'Effect of rosary prayer and yoga mantras on autonomic cardiovascular rhythms: Comparative study.' *BMJ (Clinical research ed.) 323*, 7327, 1446–1449.

Elliott, S. (2005). *The New Science of Breath.* Richardson, TX: Coherence Publishing.

Elliott, S. (2008). *Coherent Breathing: The Definitive Method.* Richardson, TX: Coherence Publishing.

Elliott, S. (2021). *Coherent Breathing.* Accessed on 15/9/2021 at: https://coherentbreathing.com.

Kiesel, K., Rhodes, T., Mueller, J., Waninger, A. and Butler, R. (2017). 'Development of a screening protocol to identify individuals with dysfunctional breathing.' *International Journal of Sports Physical Therapy 12*, 5, 774–786.

Lundberg, J. A. (1999). 'Nasal nitric oxide in man.' *Thorax*, 947–952.

McKeown, P. (2021a). *The Breathing Cure.* Galway: OxyAt Books.

McKeown, P. (2021b). *Wellness After Covid Symposium.* 29 May 2021.

Nestor, J. (2020). *Breath: The New Science of a Lost Art.* London: Penguin.

Rothenberg, R. (2020). *Restoring Prana.* London: Singing Dragon.

Schwerdtfeger, A. R., Schwarz, G., Pfurtscheller, K., Thayer, J. F., Jarczok, M. N. and Pfurtscheller, G. (2020). 'Heart rate variability (HRV): From brain death to resonance breathing at 6 breaths per minute.' *Clinical Neurophysiology 131*, 3, 676–693.

Singh, U. P. (2017). 'Evidence-based role of hypercapnia and exhalation phase in vagus nerve stimulation.' *Journal of Yoga and Physical Therapy*, 276.

Spicuzza, L., Gabutti, A., Porta, C., Montano, N. and Bernardi, L. (2000). 'Yoga and chemoreflex response to hypoxia and hypercapnia.' *Lancet 356*, 9240, 1495–1496. Erratum in: *Lancet 356*, 9241, 1612.

Stiles, M. (2021). *The Yogasutras of Patanjali.* Newburyport, MA: Weiser.

Streeter, C. C., Gerbarg, P. L., Brown, R. P., Scott, T. M., *et al.* (2020). 'Thalamic gamma aminobutyric acid level changes in major depressive disorder after a 12-week Iyengar yoga and coherent breathing intervention.' *Journal of Alternative and Complementary Medicine 26*, 3, 190–197.

Streeter, C. C., Gerbarg, P. L., Whitfield, T. H., Owen, L., *et al.* (2017). 'Treatment of major depressive disorder with Iyengar yoga and coherent breathing: A randomized controlled dosing study.' *Journal of Alternative and Complementary Medicine 23*, 3, 201–207.

CHAPTER 5

The Yoga4Health Protocol

Teach what is inside you, not as it applies to you,
but as it applies to the one in front of you.

Saying attributed to T. Krishnamacharya

The protocol is delivered by expert yoga teachers, skilled at creating a safe and non-competitive practice space. In addition, since YIHA achieved accreditation from the PCI, Yoga4Health teachers have benefited from the recognition within the NHS that they are part of the professional healthcare network, and this includes Link Workers and health coaches.

Each Yoga4Health programme cohort is made up of 5–15 students. Everyone begins the class together in chairs, and patients can continue in a chair if they are wheelchair users or have medical reasons that prevent them from moving down to the floor. Chair and mat instructions are given simultaneously, and as far as possible, chair versions of practices reflect the same work being done on the floor.

All practices are meant to be gentle, and modifications are offered to meet patient needs. For more physically able patients, progression is offered (see below), including variations and holding stretches for longer or in a deeper way. It is important that patients receive an individualized and appropriate level of physical challenge that is within their capabilities. If there is not enough rigour, this will lead to boredom and fail to maximize the many benefits of increased physical activity.

Yoga4Health teachers gather a great deal of information about each patient's medical history and health, and closely observe patients and their breath as they practise, offering advice and sometimes subtle physical adjustment if a patient has given their consent.

Although this book can be a helpful guide, nothing can replace the "live" experience of participating in a class with a Yoga4Health teacher and other students. In fact, without connection, it is not social prescribing. However, we recognized that, for a variety of reasons (such as geographical location or having missed a session and wanting to catch up), practising in isolation does happen. For this reason, YIHA has made all ten weeks of the programme available on the YIHA YouTube channel. We recommend that anyone reading this book who wishes to try the practices on their own access the free videos of the ten weekly classes (and the home-practice videos in between each session) rather than attempting to practise from the images we have included in this book. When a student practises on their own, they may not have all the background knowledge necessary to ensure they are doing the correct version of each practice that best meets their needs, as there are several to choose from. The risks are low but ought to be acknowledged.

The protocol was designed for patients who fall into the five referral categories described earlier. This protocol may not be suitable for the needs of those who fall outside these categories or fall into the exclusionary criteria. A patient may meet all referral criteria but have, for example, a hip replacement. Through their training, the Yoga4Health teacher will know how to guide movements in postures, like knees to chest, to keep this practice suitable and safe. This means that patients who are not in the exclusionary criteria but have additional issues not specifically mentioned in the inclusionary criteria can join.

To ensure safety, we recommend that anyone wishing to practise the Yoga4Health sequence consult their doctor about the suitability of the programme for them. We also urge everyone to listen to their bodies and breath while practising and apply the principle of self-care; namely, if anything does not feel right or interrupts the breath, they should release gently from that practice. Yoga practice should be undertaken without strain and within comfortable limits. No one should push into pain or significant discomfort. We advise everyone to follow the instructions for each practice and always be led by their breath.

Anyone using this book to practise the protocol does so at their own risk, which we have aimed to minimize as much as possible.

PSYCHO-EDUCATION

Every practice begins with a talk and discussion about that week's theme and the focus for the practice. In the table on p.190, we have included details about weekly themes.

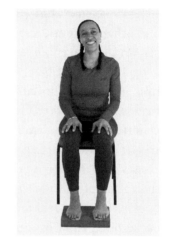

INITIAL BREATHING PRACTICE

The next segment of the class consists of learning and practising that week's breathwork. Details of the weekly breathing practices are in Chapter 4 and in the table on page 190. Students may access breathing videos on new techniques via YIHA's website.

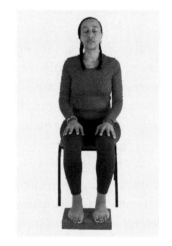

The Initial Seated Sequence –
Done by All Students

1. Inhale, spread arms wide, release shoulders. Exhale, palms together. Repeat x5 with breath-led movement.

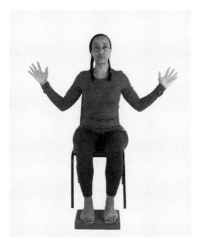 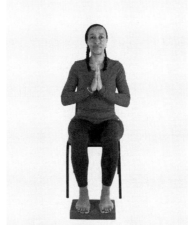

2. Inhale, raise arms from side, palms up. Turn the palms. Exhale, lower arms. Turn palms. Repeat x5 with breath-led movement.

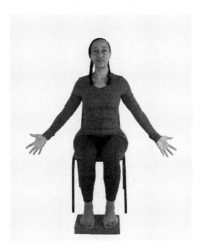 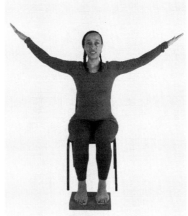

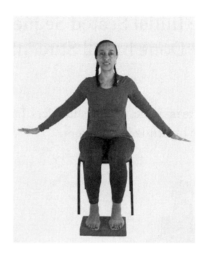

3. Mobilization:

   a. Shoulder rolls x3. Inhale, roll shoulders forward and up, and exhale, roll them back and down.

   b. Side stretch. Inhale, reach up, and exhale to R/L sides x3. Caution: only raise arm to a comfortable height.

   c. Shoulder release. Fingers to the tops of the shoulders and circle the elbows with the breath to release shoulder joint and shoulder girdle x3.

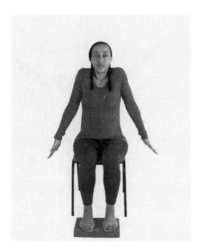
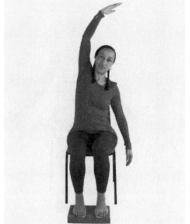

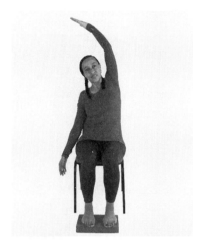 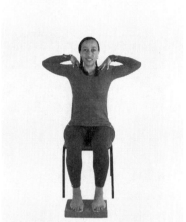

4. Neck stretch. Take the head forwards and rest the hand behind the head (do not pull). If no neck problems, rotate head gently to look towards outside of opposite thigh, 5 breaths each side.

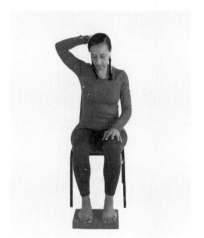 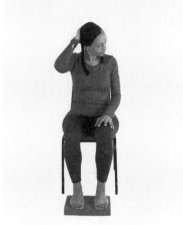

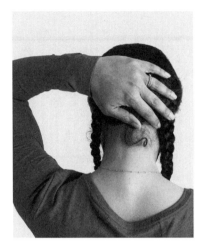 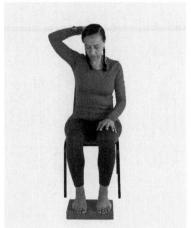

5. Seated twist. Inhale, sit tall, and exhale, rotate to the right, turning head and shoulders. Hold for 3 breaths. Inhale, turn head only back towards room and take 2 breaths. Release and repeat on left side.

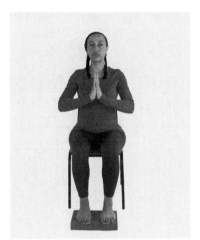 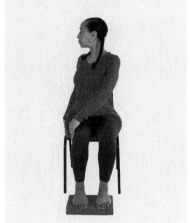

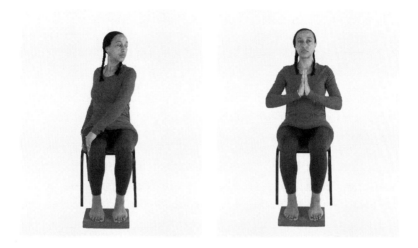

6. Opening the spine. Take hands behind the back or hold the sides of the chair. Lift the chest and take 5 slow breaths. Do not tip the head back; keep the neck long. Release into a soft forward bend for 5 breaths.

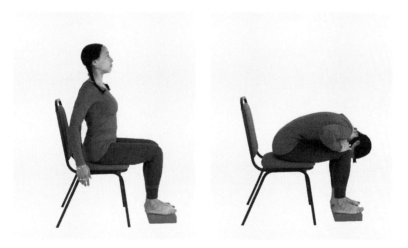

Physical Practice Continues in a Chair or on a Yoga Mat

Progression = a more challenging version of practice for more physically able patients only, or for later weeks in the protocol if appropriate to the needs of the group.

Important note: Patients working from the mat must place a folded blanket under the back of the head to maintain length in the neck. The forehead should be level with, or slightly higher than, the chin. For all kneeling practices, a thick folded blanket or cushion should be placed under the knees. For those with knee problems, follow one of the non-weight-bearing versions of modified practice.

The following sequence is available to download from https://library.jkp.com/redeem using the voucher code RZNUKLY

Mat Practice

1. Transition to the floor. Take a few breaths in this new position.

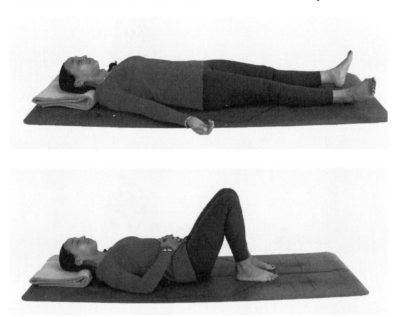

2. Inhale, slow and low, and exhale, navel to spine, to activate the core. Feel the downward movement with your palms.

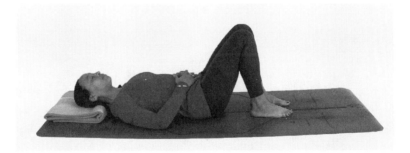

3. Long inhale, with soft arms overhead (or wherever is comfortable) to open the shoulders. Long exhale, bring the arms back to the belly and draw in the abdominal muscles x5.

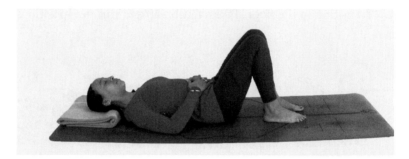

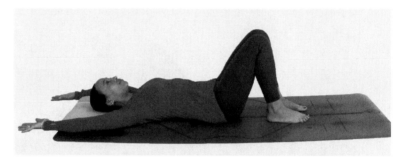

4. Circle into back of pelvis with knees and feet together to release the lower back/sacrum area, three rotations in each direction. *Progression*: Same practice without arms, demanding additional abdominal strength.

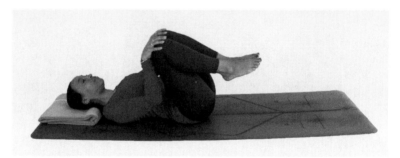

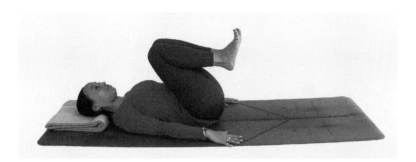

5. Hold shin or thigh (or use belt) in semi-supine and rotate, flex/ point ankle, R/L sides. Hold right shin/thigh with arms straight, left leg bent. Draw thigh in during exhale x3. Repeat left side. *Progression*: Straighten bent leg x3, R/L sides. Knees to chest and rock to counterpose.

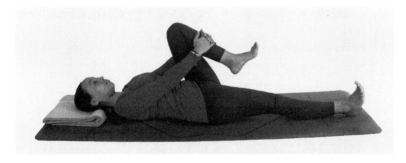

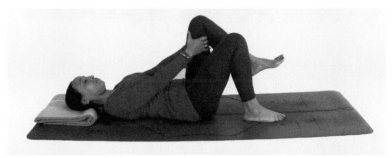

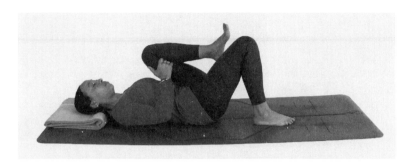

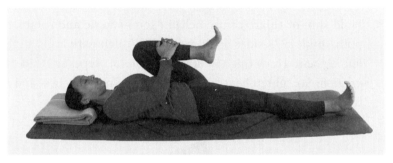

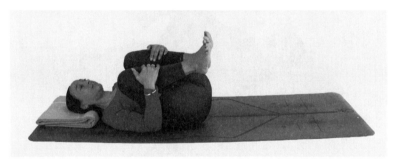

6. Exhaling, lift tailbone by contracting abdominal muscles only. Release on inhale x3–5.

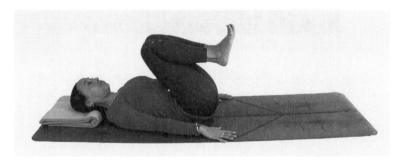

7. Wide slow knee circles coordinated with the breath to open the hips – both directions x5.

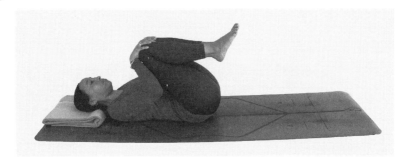

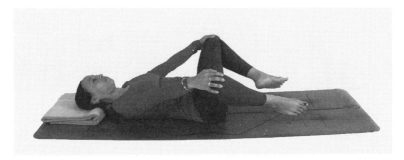

8. Inhale, full body stretch, engaging as many muscles as possible. Exhale, relax completely x5.

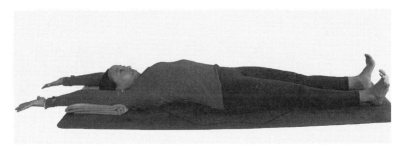

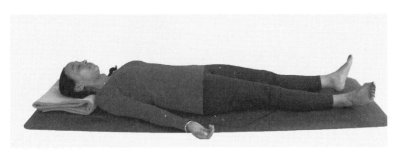

9. Hold full body stretch for 5 breaths. Release into softness for 5 breaths.

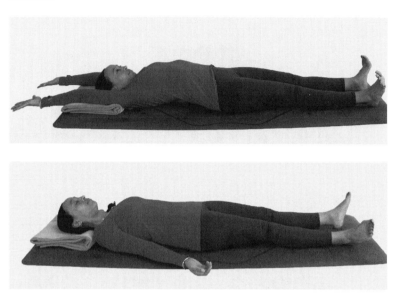

10. Dynamic supine twist. Arms away from the body at shoulder height or bend elbows (as shown here). Shoulders back and down, palms up. Feet hip width apart. Inhale centre and exhale x3 into twist, R/L sides.

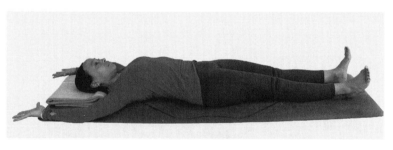

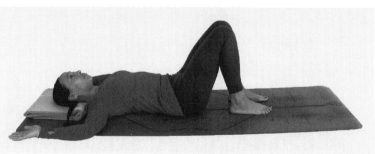

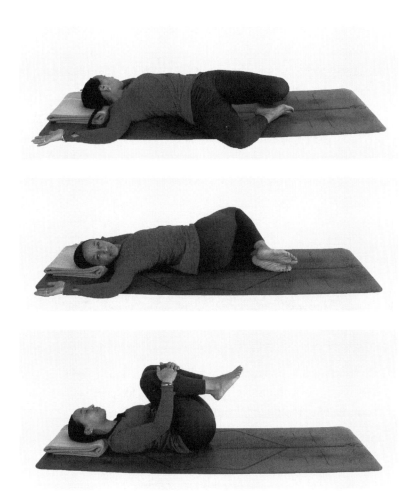

11. Held twist x5 breaths, R/L sides. Hug in knees to counterpose.

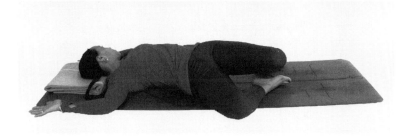

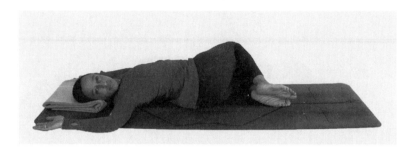

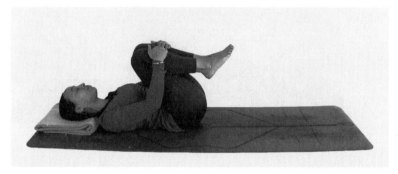

12. Cross-crawl and hamstring stretch. Inhale, left arm, right leg. Exhale, semi-supine. Inhale, right arm, left leg. Exhale, semi-supine x3 rounds. Hug in knees to counterpose.

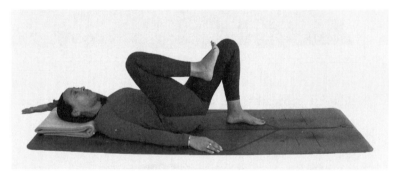

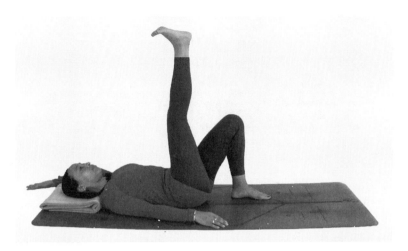

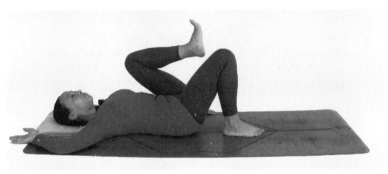

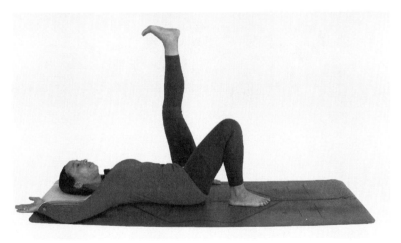

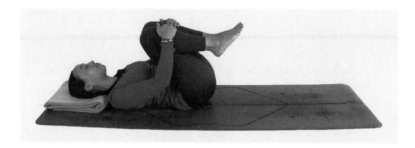

13. Pelvic tilts with breath. Inhale, lift front of pelvis slightly, and exhale, tuck tail under, engaging pelvic floor x5.

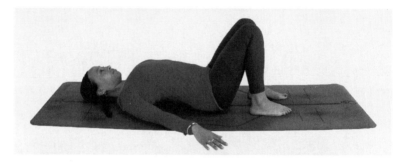

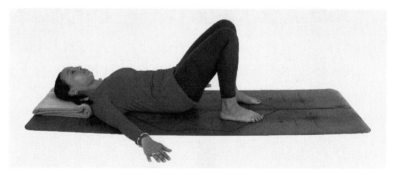

14. Dynamic bridge pose. Remove any padding under head. Inhale, lift hips (a little higher on each lift), and exhale, roll spine back down to the mat x5. Keep abdomen drawn in. Counterpose with knees to chest.

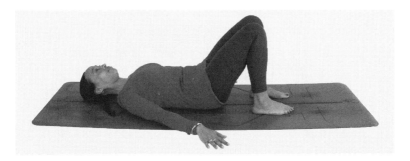

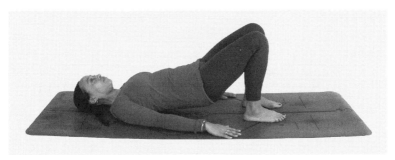

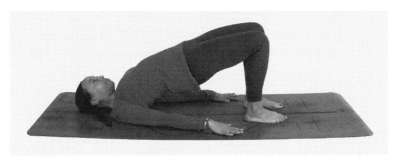

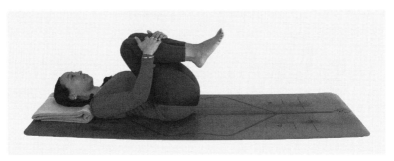

15. Held bridge pose. Inhale, lift into pose with feet hip width apart and hold for 5 breaths. *Progression*: Link hands under back and stretch arms. Hug in knees to counterpose.

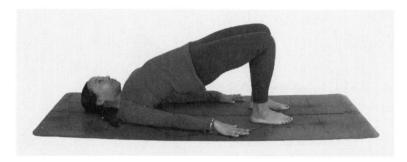

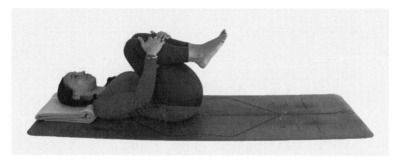

16. Dynamic hamstring stretch with belt. Bend right leg on inhale, and stretch on exhale x5. After last exhale, hold static stretch right side x5 breaths. Relax and observe effects of stretch *before* repeating left side.

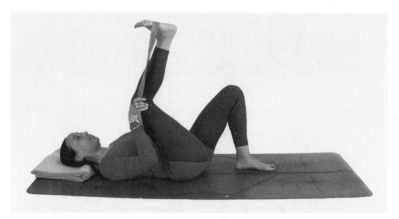

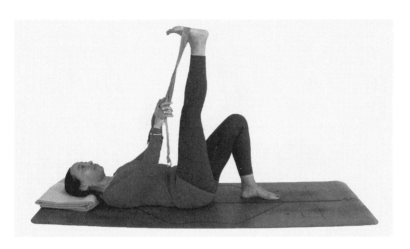

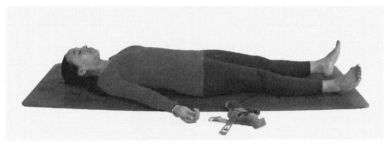

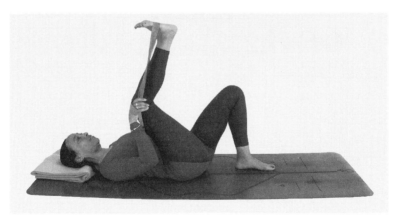

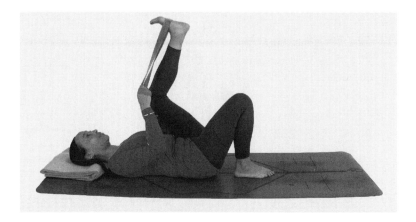

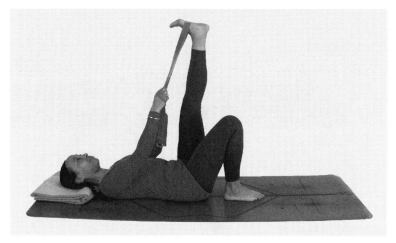

17. Thread the needle hip stretch. Patients with knee problems, tight hips or lower back discomfort should perform the most modified version. Release knee to side, or place right foot onto left thigh above the knee. Flex right ankle to protect the knee. *Progression*: Keep left foot closer to the body for stronger hip opening. Raise left leg and hold left thigh for deeper expression of the pose. 5 breaths R/L sides. Hug in knees to counterpose.

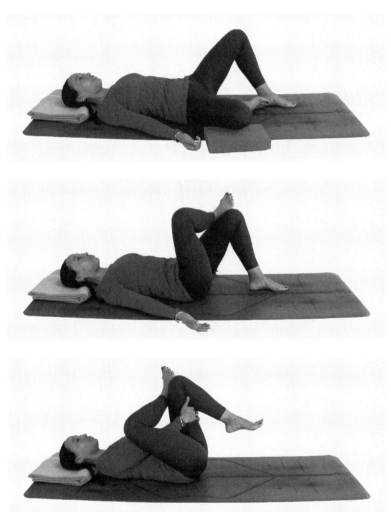

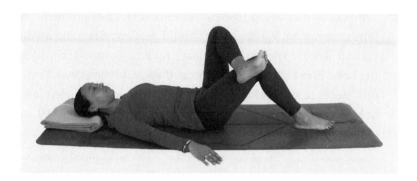

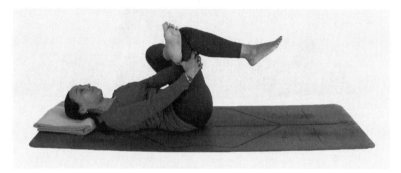

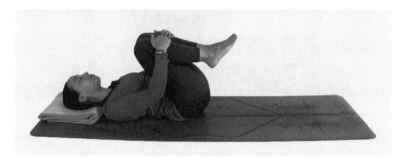

18. Cat pose. Pad knees and place hands slightly in front of shoulders or on chair (for knee, wrist or shoulder problems, do the chair-supported version shown on page 164). Inhale, release the spine into backbend and lift the head slightly. Exhale, arch the back towards the ceiling, allowing the head to relax down x5. Release into resting pose.

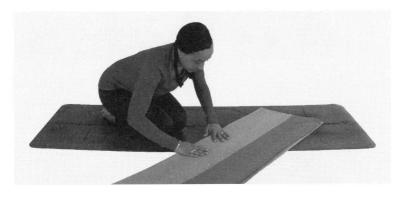

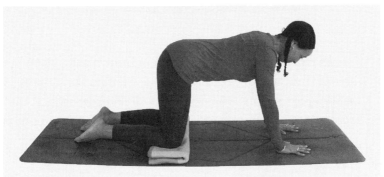

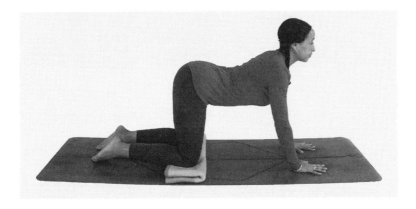

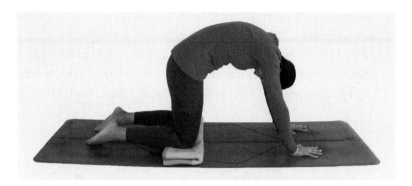

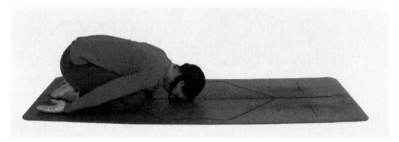

19. Forearm sphinx (backbend). Lie on your front, make a pillow for the forehead (on hands or yoga block). After a few breaths come up onto forearms, elbows forward of shoulders (or under for more flexibility). Front of hips remain on the mat x5 breaths. Release into resting pose.

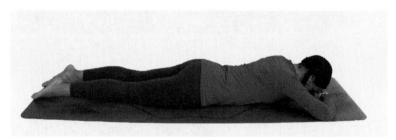

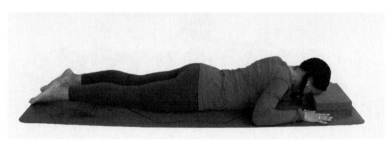

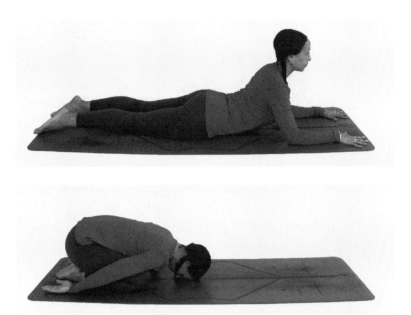

20. Back strengthening. Take the arms wide and rest forehead on mat/ yoga block. Inhale, lift head and upper chest using the back muscles only, and exhale, lower x3. *Progression*: Hold lifted position for a further 3 breaths. Release into resting pose.

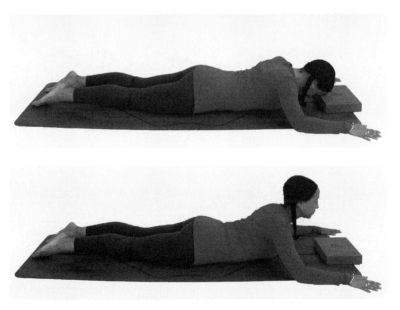

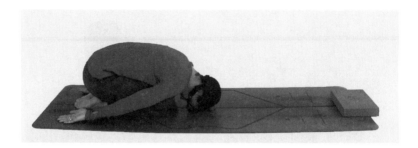

21. Glute strengthening. Rest forehead on mat/yoga block. Inhale, lift the straight right leg, and exhale, bring it down. Inhale, lift the left leg, and exhale, bring it down x3, R/L sides. When lifting the leg, keep front of hips pressing into the mat. Take release pose.

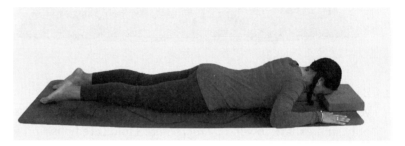

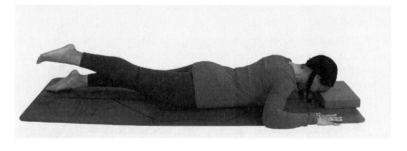

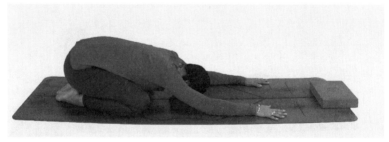

22. Dynamic downward facing dog. From all fours (knees padded), tuck toes and inhale to lengthen spine. Exhale, lift the hips high, stay on toes/balls of feet, knees bent. Inhale, hold position and lengthen spine further. Exhale, lower knees. Repeat x3–5. For those with medical reasons not to invert, do the chair-supported versions on page 169. Take resting pose at end or between poses.

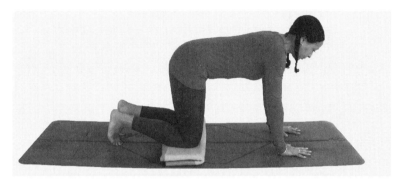

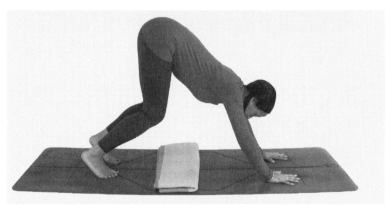

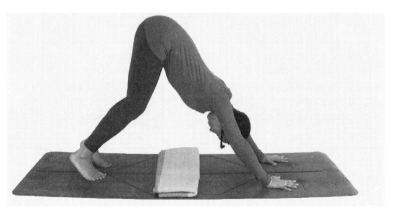

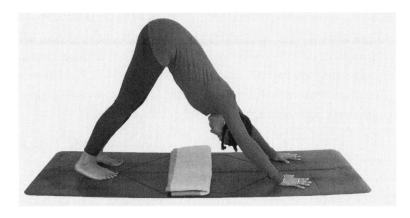

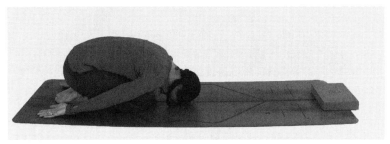

23. Downward facing dog. Hold downward facing dog x5 breaths. You may also "walk the dog" by gently stretching alternate legs on an exhale. Take resting pose.

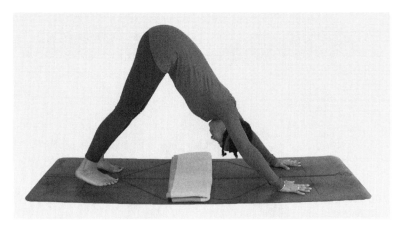

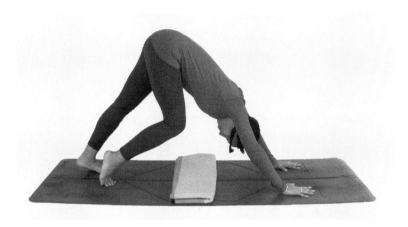

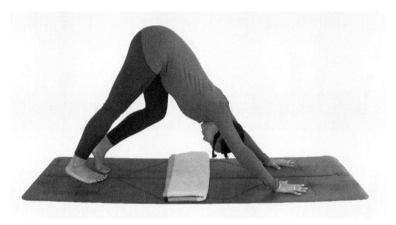

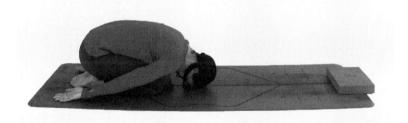

24. Stand in mountain pose, feet hip width apart. Take a few breaths here, feeling the touch of the feet on the ground. Shrug shoulders, rotate wrists, extend fingers and make soft fists x3–5.

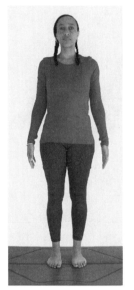
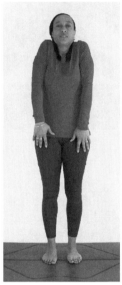
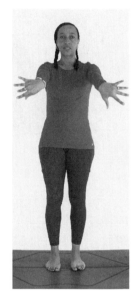

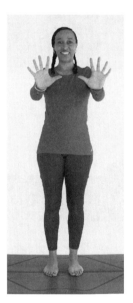
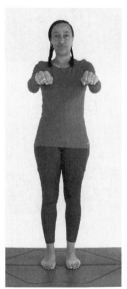

25. Extend arms to the sides and sweep up on inhale, draw palms down past the heart on exhale. Repeat x5, lifting toes on inhale and relaxing them on exhale, and then lifting the heels on inhale and releasing them on exhale.

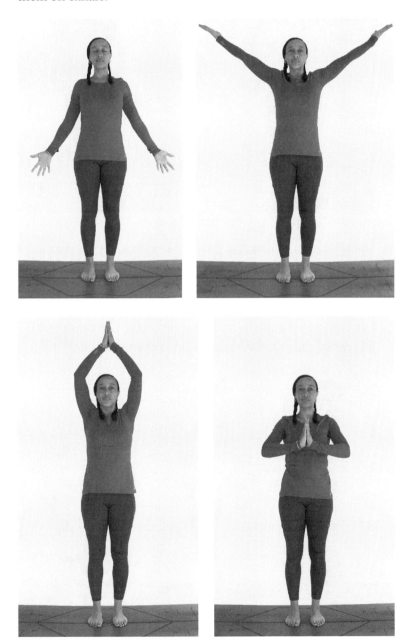

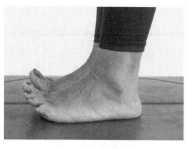

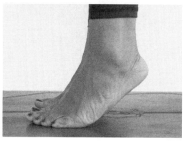

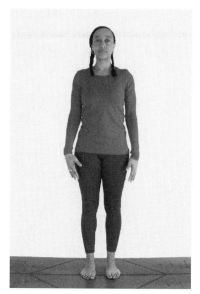

26. Sun salutation. A dynamic series of interwoven yoga postures that stretch the body and support cardiovascular, respiratory and lymphatic health. Each pose is done either on an inhale or exhale; no pose is held.

Inhale, sweep the arms out to the sides and up overhead. Exhale, and fold forwards from the hips, bending the knees.

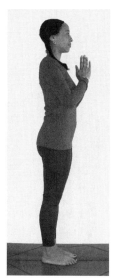

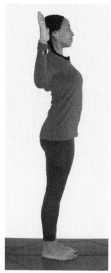

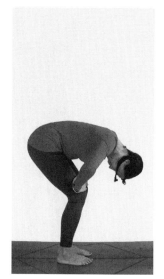

27. Inhale, engage back muscles to flatten the back or place forearms on thighs. Exhale, fold forwards again. *Progression*: On inhale, hover the hands for additional strengthening work.

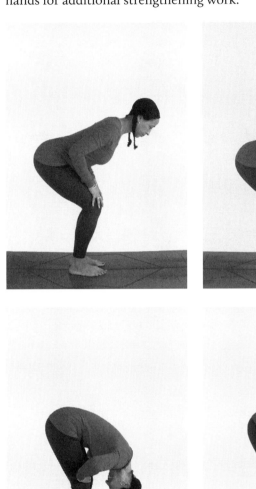

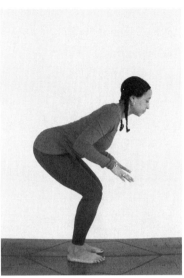

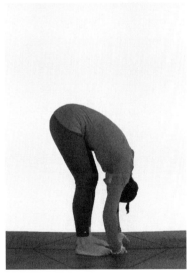

28. Inhale, bend the knees and come up with a flat back, sweeping the arms out to the sides and up. Exhale, draw the palms down to the centre of the chest.

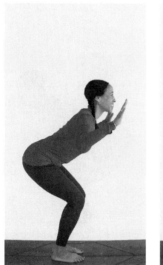 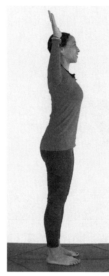 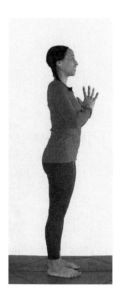

29. Inhale, reach up from the centre of the body to a comfortable position with palms touching. Try not to lift the shoulders. Exhale, sway right. Inhale, reach up. Exhale, palms together in front of heart.

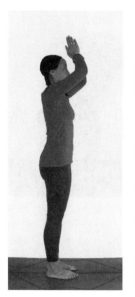 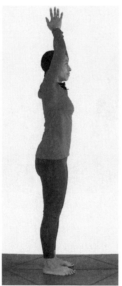 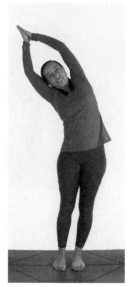

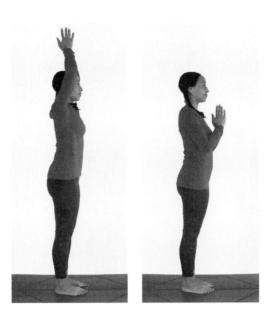

30. Inhale, reach up. Exhale, sway left. Inhale, reach up. Exhale palms in front of heart.

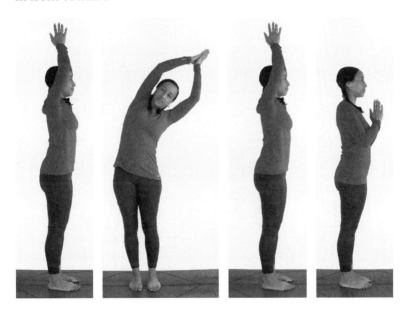

31. *Repeat sun salutations up to five times.*

32. Dynamic warrior 1. Keep feet hip width apart and back foot hardly turned out. Inhale to bend knee into lunge and take arms wide, shoulders released. Exhale, return palms together and straighten leg x5 R/L sides.

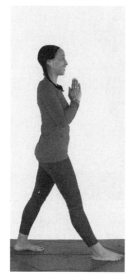
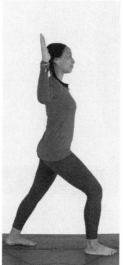
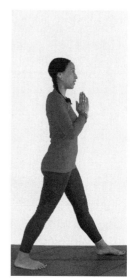

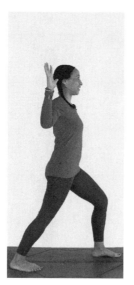
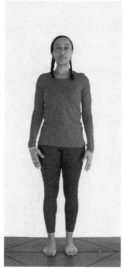

33. Dynamic warrior 2. Step feet apart a comfortable distance and hold hips steady. Turn the right leg and foot out 70–80 degrees (according to your own hip range of motion). Palms together. Inhale, turn head, extend arms and lunge right leg (knee tracks second toe). Exhale, return to starting position x5, R/L sides.

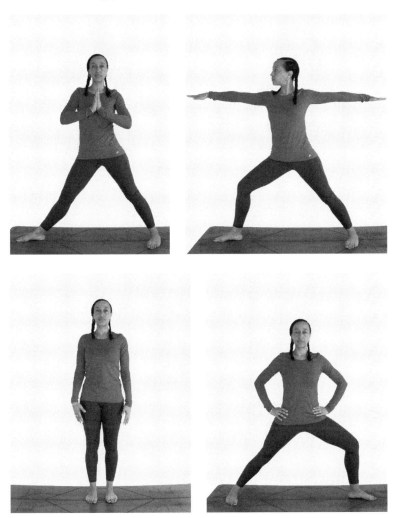

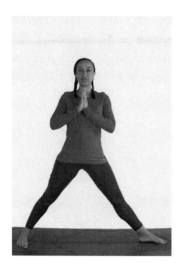

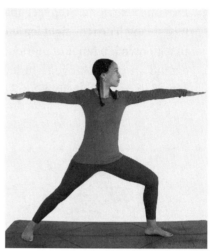

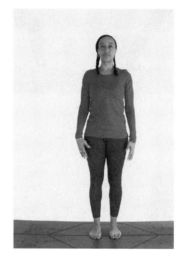

34. Dynamic heron balance. Start in mountain pose. Inhale, lift the arms and come onto the toes of the right foot. Exhale, release down. Switch legs with each breath and progress to lifting and lowering the foot to and from the mat x5, R/L sides. If you have balance issues, use a chair or wall for support. *Progression*: In later weeks, patients may move on to holding the raised leg for 3–5 breaths.

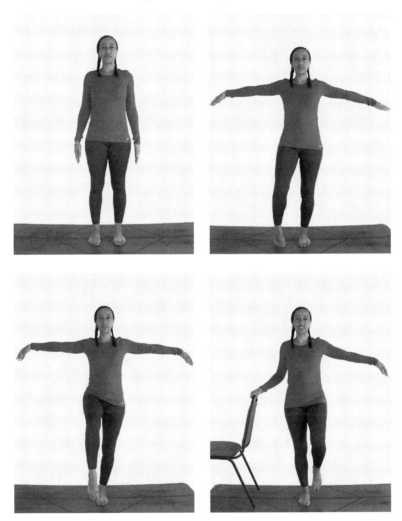

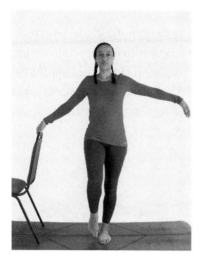
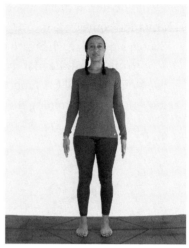

35. Tree pose. Turn out leg at the hip and raise heel. Progress to bringing one foot on top of the other or foot up to shin. *Progression*: Foot above knee for full position. Arms to side or overhead. 5 breaths, R/L sides. Use a chair or wall for stability if needed.

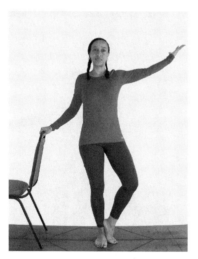
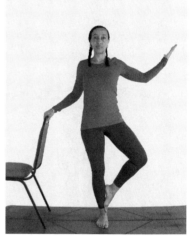

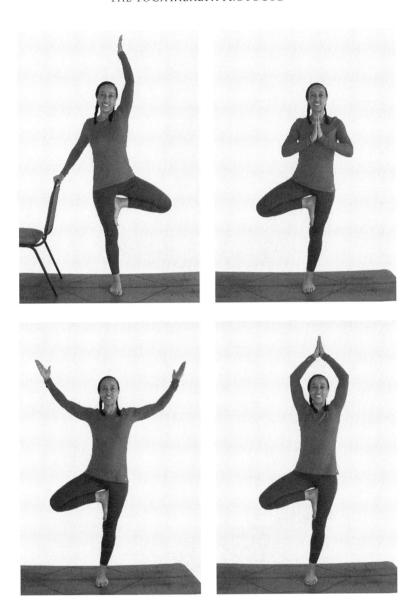

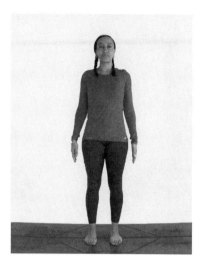

Note: Heron balance is taught in the first half of the course and tree balance in the second half, with progression towards held balances if suitable. However, either balance may be taught on any week to meet patient needs.

36. Mild inversion. Rest the legs on the chair, yoga block under the hips and head supported on a blanket. 10 breaths.

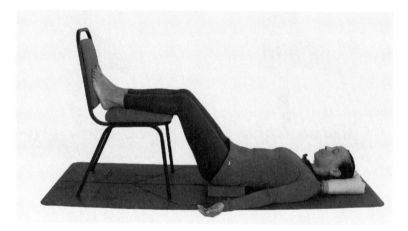

37. Relaxation. Find a comfortable pose using any available supports if needed, or take semi-supine with knees together. Listen to a recorded Yoga4Health relaxation (ten available to download).

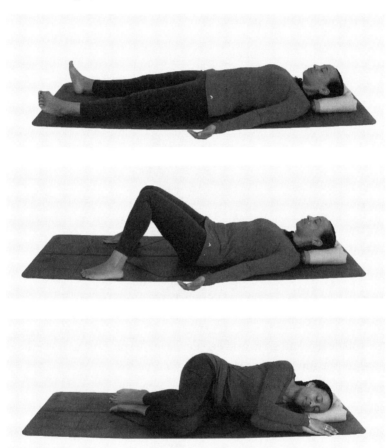

Chair Practice

1. Sit quietly with your breath.

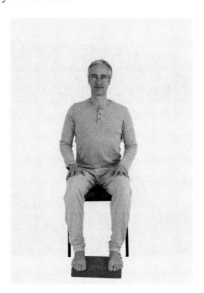

2. Inhale low and slow, and exhale, navel to spine, to activate the core. Feel the inward movement with your palms.

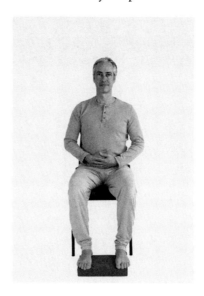

3. Long inhale, raise soft arms to a comfortable height. Long exhale, bring the arms back to the belly and draw in the abdominal muscles x5.

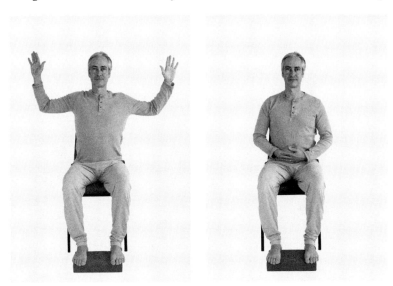

4. Circle the upper body, feeling the shift in weight around the base of the pelvis. Keep core engaged.

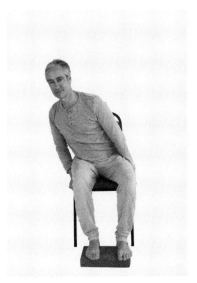
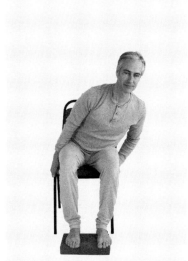

5. Hold shin or thigh (or use belt) and rotate, flex/point ankle, R/L sides. Hold shin or thigh (or use belt) and draw in thigh on exhale x3–5, R/L sides. Fold forwards to release.

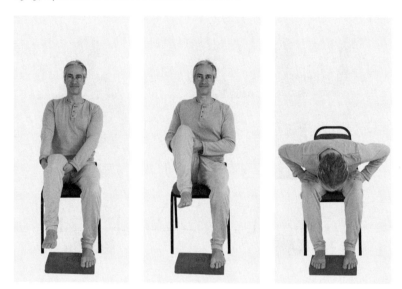

6. Draw up pelvic floor on exhale, keeping the rest of the body relaxed. Release pelvic floor during inhale x5.

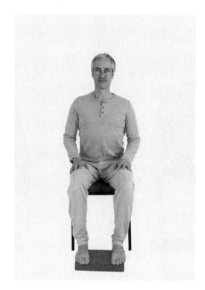

7. Hold one knee or shin at a time and do wide slow knee circles coordinated with the breath x3, R/L sides.

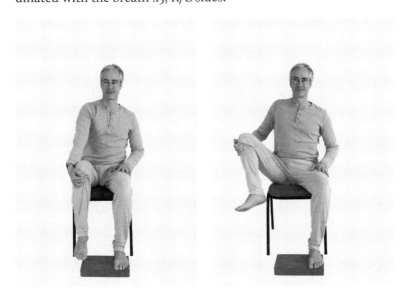

8. Inhale, reach up and engage as many muscles as possible. Exhale, relax x5.

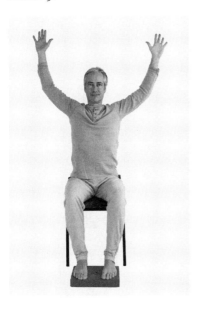 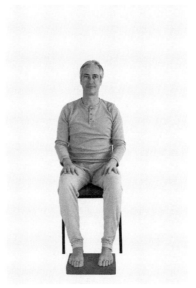

9. Hold raised arm stretch for up to 2–5 breaths. Release into softness for 5 breaths.

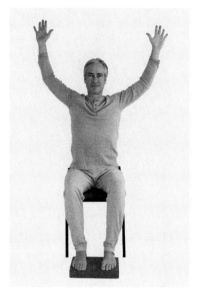
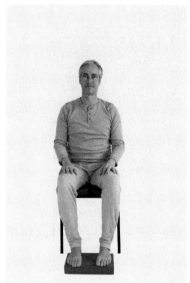

10. Dynamic twist. Inhale, palms together, lengthen up. Exhale, turn shoulders and head in opposite directions, release palms down. Inhale to centre, palms together, and exhale x3 into twist, R/L sides.

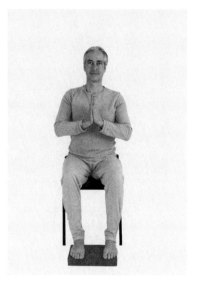
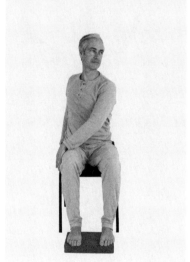

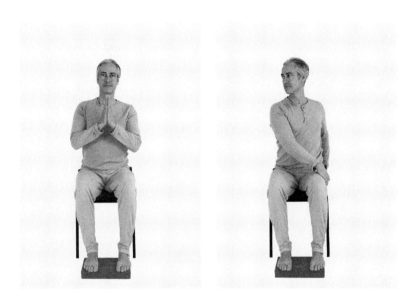

11. Inhale, lengthen spine, and exhale into twist. Turn head in opposite direction and hold posture x5 breaths, R/L sides. Forward fold to counterpose. *Progression*: Turn sideways on chair and turn to hold back of chair to support a deeper twist.

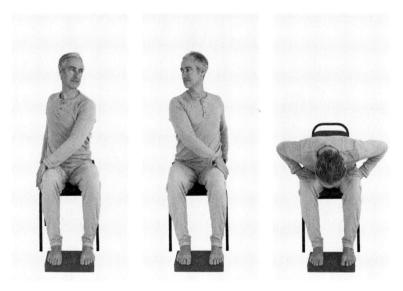

12. Cross-crawl and hamstring stretch. Inhale, left arm, right leg. Exhale, release. Inhale, right arm, left leg. Exhale, release x3 rounds.

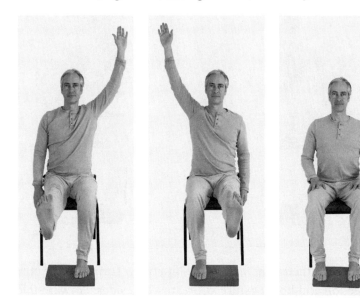

13. Pelvic tilts with breath. Inhale, front of pelvis moves forwards slightly, and exhale, tuck tail under, engaging pelvic floor x5.

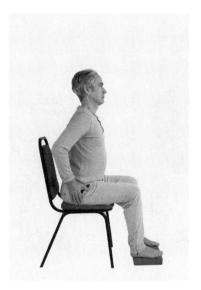
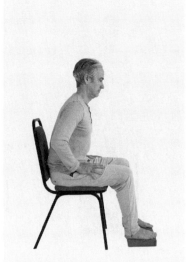

14. Dynamic backbend. Inhale, open chest, and exhale, release back to neutral x5. Counterpose with forward fold.

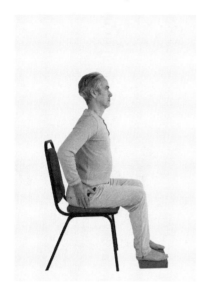 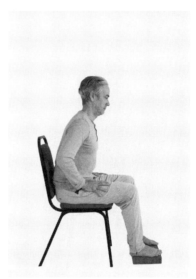

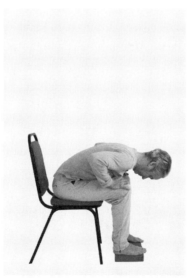

15. Held backbend. Inhale, open chest and hold x5 breaths. Keep back of neck long. Counterpose with forward fold.

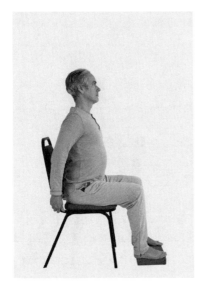 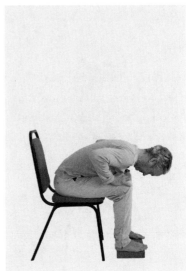

16. Dynamic hamstring stretch with belt. Bend right leg on inhale, and stretch on exhale x5. After last exhale hold static stretch right side x5 breaths. Relax and observe effects of stretch *before* repeating left side.

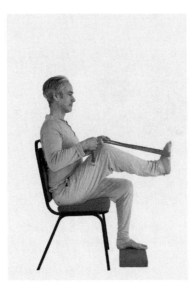 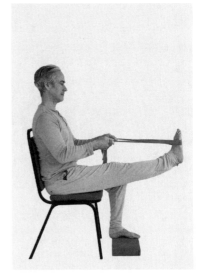

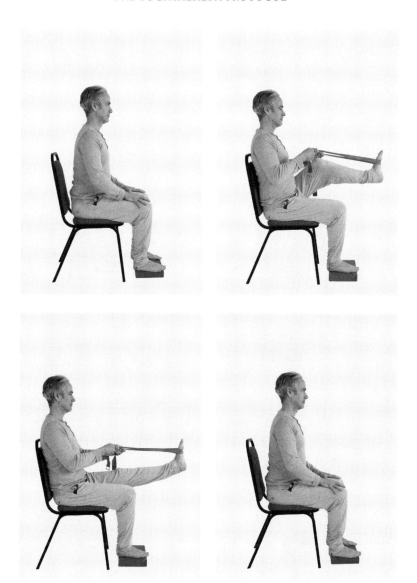

17. Thread the needle hip stretch. Place right foot on an appropriate support and release knee. Flex right ankle to protect knee. *Progression*: Place right ankle on left thigh if hips/knees allow. 5 breaths, R/L sides.

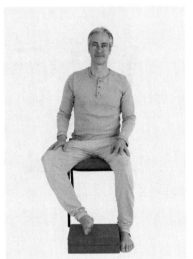 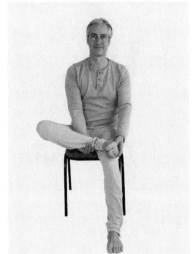

18. Cat pose. From a chair, inhale and open the spine, sliding hands towards hips. Exhale, round the back and engage the abdominals, sliding hands towards knees. For those who can stand with support, use back of a chair x5.

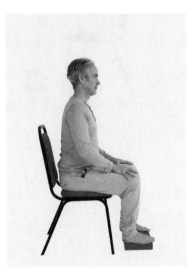 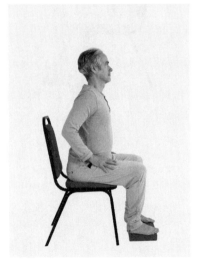

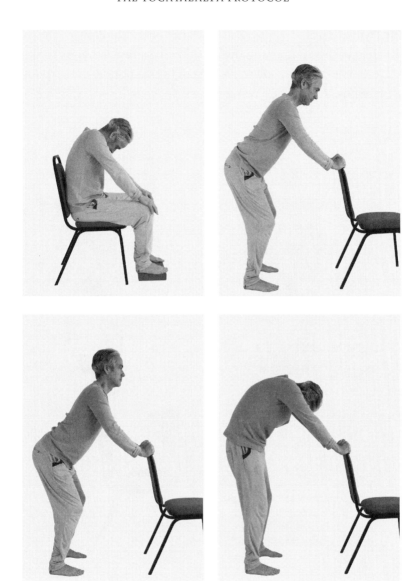

19. Dynamic seated sphinx. Raise the arms on inhale, drawing the shoulders back and opening the chest. Exhale, return hands to thighs. If kneeling to use chair, pad knees for supported static sphinx x5 breaths. Release into resting pose.

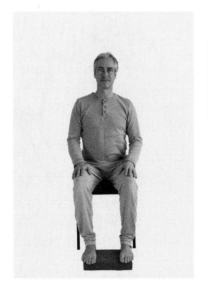
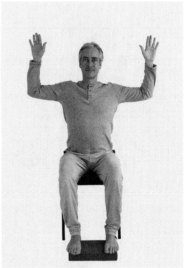

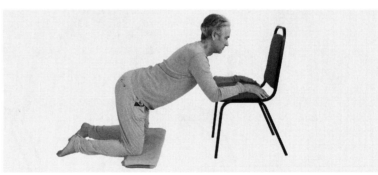

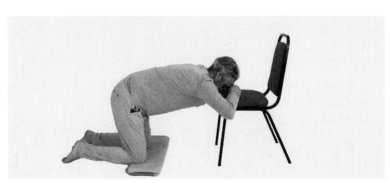

20. Back strengthening. Lean forward onto the thighs and use back muscles to arch and release the spine with the breath x3 breaths. *Progression*: Hover the hands to increase back muscle strengthening. Hold for 3 breaths and exhale to release pose. Alternatively, pad knees and use a chair to lift and lower elbows with breath.

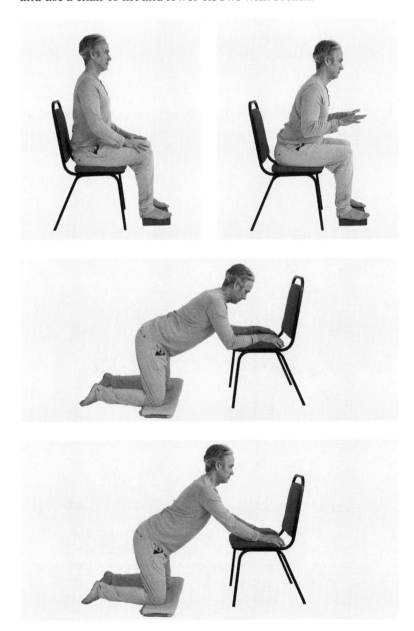

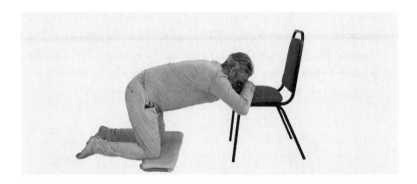

21. Glute strengthening. Inhale, contract glutes, and exhale, release x3, R/L sides. For those who can kneel, pad knees and raise alternate bent legs with breath x3, R/L sides. Take resting pose.

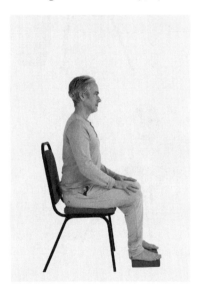 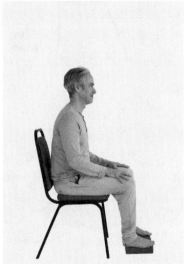

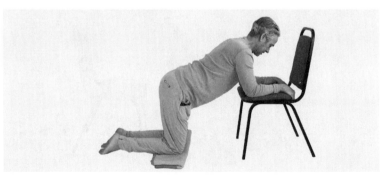

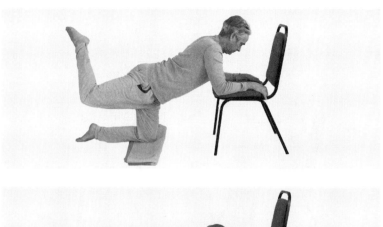

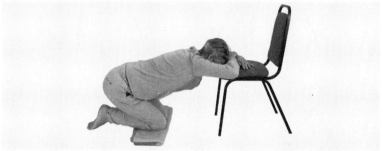

22. Dynamic downward facing dog. Inhale, lift both arms and right leg, and exhale, release. Inhale both arms and left leg, exhale release. Repeat up to x5. Take resting pose. *Progression*: If you can stand, use the back of the chair. Inhale, look forwards, and exhale, take downward facing dog. Inhale, hold position, and exhale, come back up. Repeat x3–5.

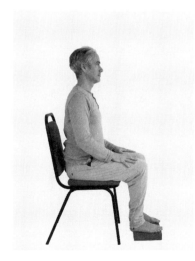
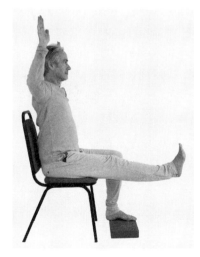

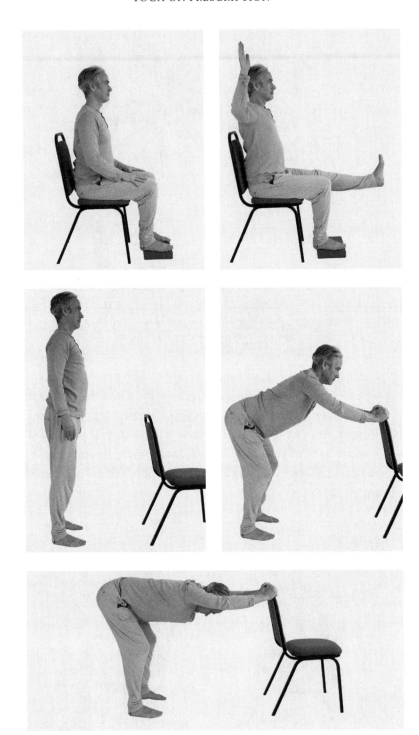

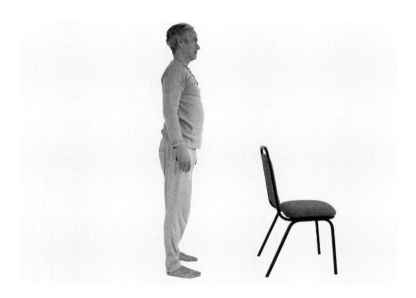

23. Downward facing dog. Hold downward facing dog x3 breaths, R/L sides. Take resting pose. Alternatively, hold the supported chair dog x5 breaths.

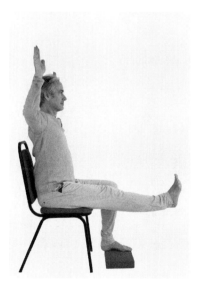
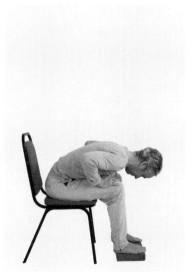

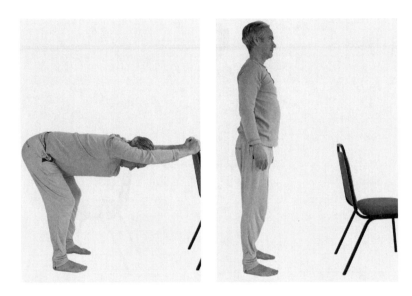

24. Sit quietly for a moment and notice how you feel. Then shrug shoulders, rotate wrists, extend fingers and make soft fists x3–5.

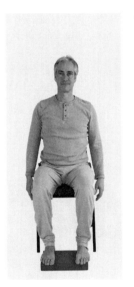 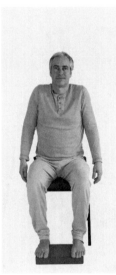 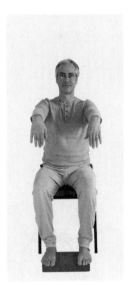

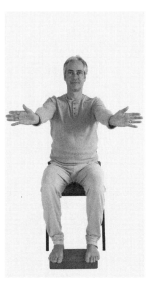 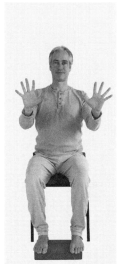 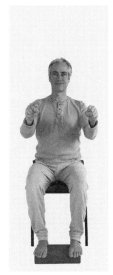

25. Extend arms to the sides and sweep up on inhale, draw palms down past the heart on exhale. Repeat x5, lifting toes on inhale and relaxing them on exhale, and lifting the heels on inhale and releasing them on exhale.

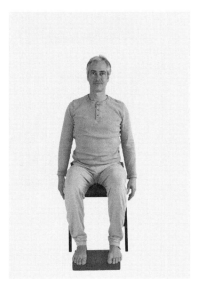 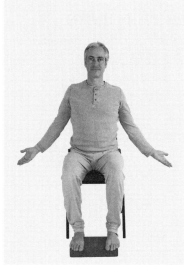

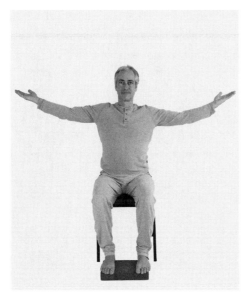

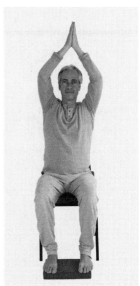

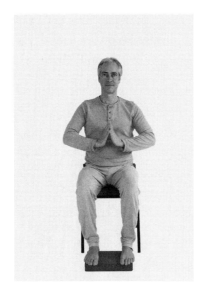

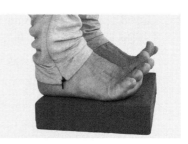

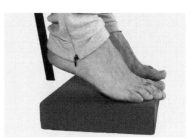

26. Sun salutations. A dynamic series of interwoven yoga postures that
stretch the body and support cardiovascular, respiratory and lymphatic health. Each pose is done either on an inhale or exhale; no
pose is held.

Inhale, sweep the arms out to the sides and up overhead. Exhale, and
fold forwards over the thighs.

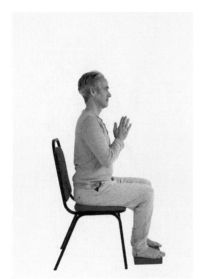
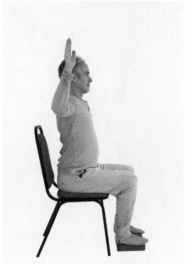

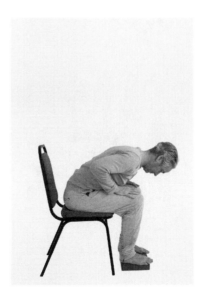

27. Inhale, engage back muscles to flatten the back. Exhale, fold forwards again. *Progression*: On inhale, hover the hands for additional strengthening work.

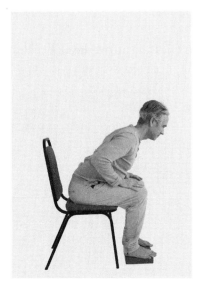 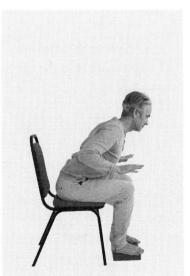

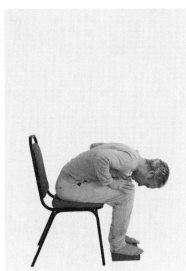

28. Inhale, come up with a flat back, sweeping the arms out to the sides and up. Exhale, draw the palms down to the centre of the chest.

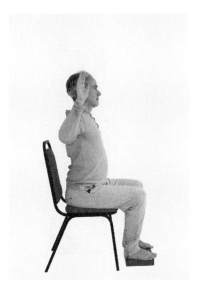 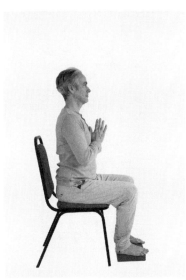

29. Inhale, reach up from the centre of the body to a comfortable position with the palms touching. Try not to lift the shoulders. Exhale, sway right. Inhale, reach up. Exhale palms together in front of heart.

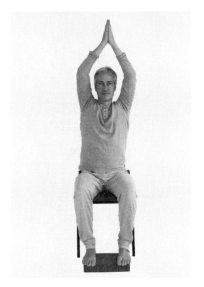 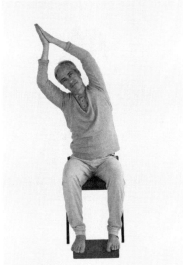

Or

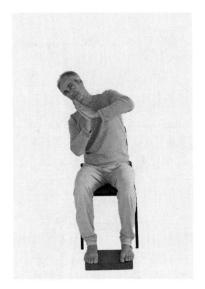
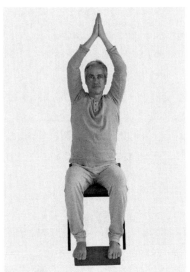

Or

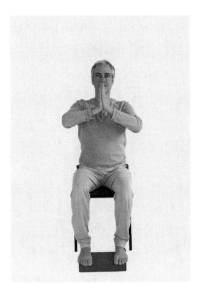
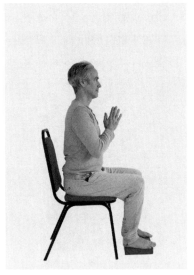

30. Inhale, reach up. Exhale, sway left. Inhale, reach up. Exhale, palms in front of heart.

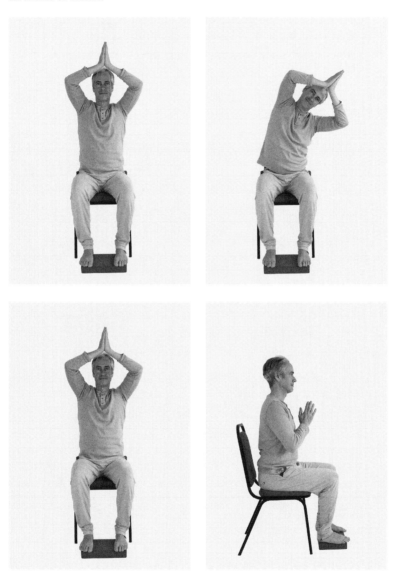

31. *Repeat sun salutations up to 5 times.*

32. Dynamic warrior 1. Take the left leg to the side and bring palms together in front of the heart. Inhale, open arms, and exhale, palms together x5, R/L sides. If you can stand, use the back of the chair, feet hip width apart and hips facing forwards. Inhale, bend the leg, and exhale, straighten x5, R/L sides.

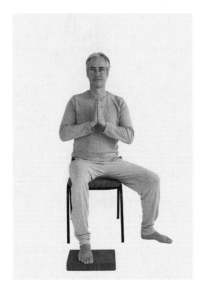
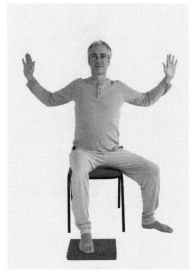
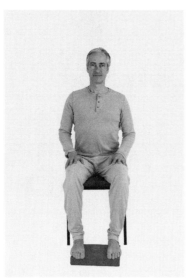
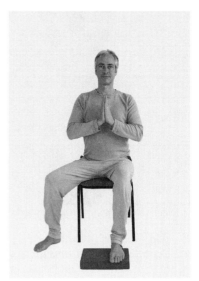

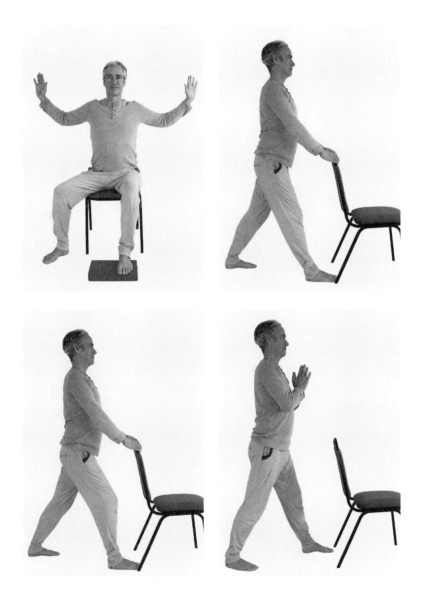

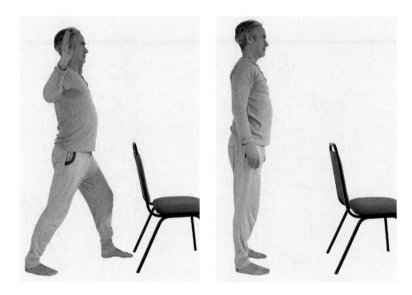

33. Dynamic warrior 2. Open right hip and turn out left leg slightly. Palms together. Inhale, turn head, extend arms. Exhale, return to starting position x5, R/L sides. Alternatively, with chair support, extend arm and bend knee on inhale. Straighten leg and draw in arm on exhale x5, R/L sides.

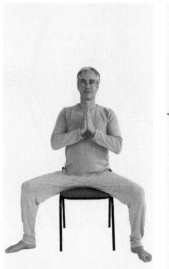

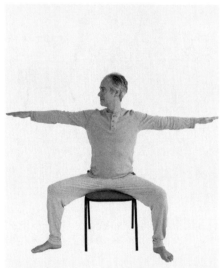

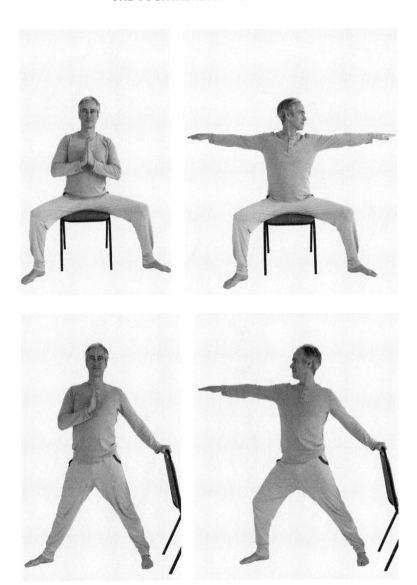

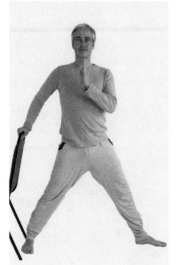
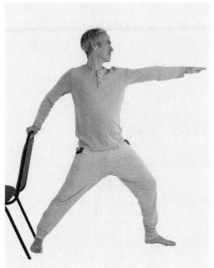

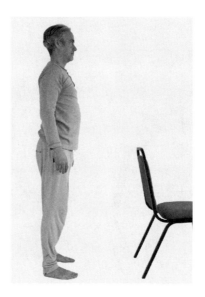

34. Dynamic heron pose. Only work in a chair if you are unable to stand. Inhale, raise soft arms to the sides and lift right leg. Exhale, lower. Continue with alternate legs and both arms. Using a chair or wall for stability, extend one arm and lift alternate legs with the breath x5, R/L sides. *Progression*: In later weeks, patients may move on to holding the raised leg for 3–5 breaths.

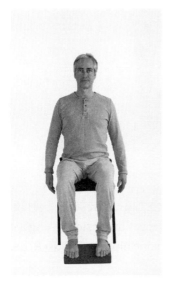
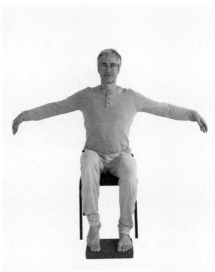

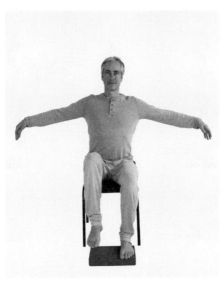

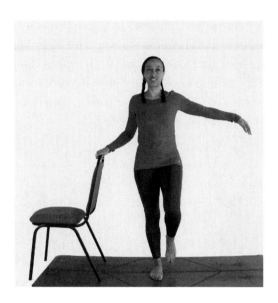

35. Tree pose. Only work in a chair if you are unable to stand. Extend both arms like tree branches, open one hip and rest the heel on the opposite ankle. Hold for 5 breaths. Repeat other side. Using a chair for stability, extend one arm and open one hip at a time x5, R/L sides.

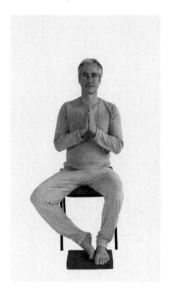

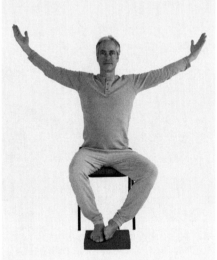

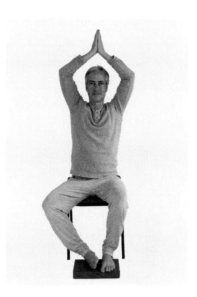

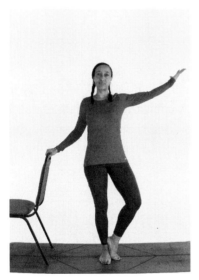
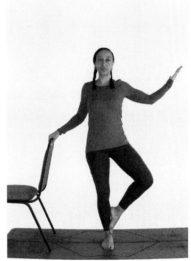

Note: Heron balance is taught in the first half of the course and tree balance in the second half, with progression towards held balances if suitable. However, either balance may be taught on any week to meet patient needs.

36. Mild inversion. Sit comfortably in the chair. If possible, raise the legs and rest on another chair, 10 breaths. *Progression*: If coming to the floor for relaxation, rest legs on chair as shown on page 152.

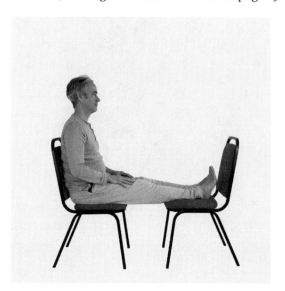

37. Relaxation. If your chair has sides you may be able to safely relax. If not, sit against a wall in case you fall asleep and fall off the chair. If remaining in a chair without sides, treat relaxation as a guided meditation. Listen to a recorded Yoga4Health relaxation (ten available to download).

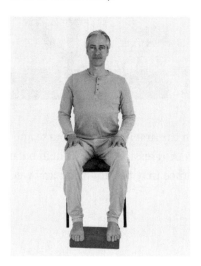 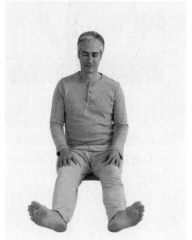

Final Breathing Practice

The week's breathing technique is further established by around 5 minutes of practice (see Chapter 4).

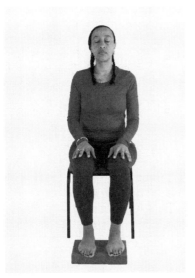 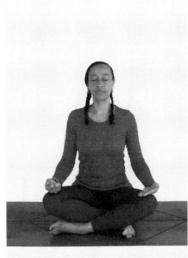

GROUP DISCUSSION

Up to 20 minutes of group discussion takes place to reflect on the class and its theme and hear about different experiences in the group (see also Chapter 1). This process of reflection can be replicated by those practising alone by taking time to write down reflections on the class in a yoga practice diary. Suggested ideas for what to reflect on are included in the table below.

PRACTISING THE TEN-WEEK PROGRAMME

The table below summarizes the content and themes of the ten-week programme and how patients develop their experience of the protocol.

Week	Theme	Breathing	Physical poses	Relaxation	Breathwork	Reflection
1	Body and breath awareness Notice where you feel your breath	Abdominal breathing/breath awareness. Noticing the breath in every pose	Follow protocol, taking modified forms of each practice	Breathing in and out of different parts of the body	General breath awareness focusing on abdominal breathing	What did you feel in your body? How was your breath?
2	Grounding Part 1 Feel the touch of the body on the ground	Breathing up and down from the ground	Follow protocol, building familiarity	Breathing up and down from the ground while releasing the body	Breathing up from the feet to the chest and exhaling back down to the feet	Do you feel more grounded? Could you direct the breath?
3	Grounding Part 2 Inhale from the ground, exhale elongated ocean breath back down to the ground	Learning ocean breath and using the long exhale to emphasize connection back down to the ground	Follow protocol, building familiarity and using the long exhale in poses	Development of breathing up and down from the ground while releasing the body	Inhale up from the soles of the feet, long ocean breath exhale back down to the ground	Has your breath changed? Does the long exhale enhance grounding?
4	Grounding Part 3 Inhale ocean breath up from the ground, exhale elongated ocean breath back down to the ground	Learning ocean breath on inhale as well as on long exhale down to the ground	Follow protocol, beginning to explore how the long exhale deepens stretches	Further development of breathing up and down from the ground while releasing the body	Inhale ocean breath up from the soles of the feet, long ocean breath exhale back down to the ground	Do you feel more in control of your breath? Has three weeks of grounding changed how you feel?

Week	Theme	Breathing	Physical poses	Relaxation	Breathwork	Reflection
5	Spaciousness Inhale, exhale, pause/space	Exploring space in the breath. Inhale ocean breath, exhale ocean breath, pause/space	Using the long exhale and pause to further deepen stretches and meditative quality of practice	Relaxation themed on finding space in the body and breath	Inhale ocean breath, creating space in the body, exhale long ocean breath and pause – notice the space in breath, body, mind	Did the pause make a difference? Does your exhale feel longer?
6	Spaciousness Notice your shoulders in every pose	Inhale ocean breath, exhale ocean breath, pause/space	Using the long exhale and pause to further deepen stretches and meditative quality of practice. Experiencing space in postures	Relaxation themed on finding space in the body and breath	Inhale ocean breath, creating space in the body, exhale long ocean breath and pause – notice the shoulders, release the shoulders	Has your practice changed to breath-led? Is there more space in your body and mind?
7	Awareness of bodily sensations Notice the sensations in the body	Inhale ocean breath, exhale ocean breath, pause/space	Noticing sensations in every pose. Further exploring depth of practice using the long exhale and pause	Relaxation focusing on sensations in every part of the body	Inhale ocean breath, exhale long ocean breath and pause – notice sensations in the body	Do you feel more aware of sensations in your body in class? In life generally?

cont.

Week	Theme	Breathing	Physical poses	Relaxation	Breathwork	Reflection
8	Balance Breathe with the chimes	Coherent Breathing: Inhaling for 6 seconds and exhaling for 6 seconds cued by the sound of the chimes or piano	Feeling a sense of balance in every practice. Using the chimes and Coherent Breathing to lead the physical practice	Relaxation moving from side to side in the body to promote balance	Coherent Breathing using the audio track. Creating balance in the breath	How did you find working with chimes? Were they too fast, too slow or just right?
9	Change Notice the beginning/end of the inhale and exhale. Notice the arising and passing of sensations	Coherent Breathing: Inhaling for 6 seconds and exhaling for 6 seconds cued by the sound of the chimes or piano	Noticing beginnings and endings in breath and postures. Moving beyond gross physical practice and deepening breath-led movement	Relaxation focusing on sensations and noticing when they pass	Coherent Breathing using the audio track. Noticing changes in the quality of our breath	Could you notice the beginning and end of your breath? Did sensations arise and pass?
10	Connection We are all breathing together; we are all connected by breath	Coherent Breathing: Inhaling for 6 seconds and exhaling for 6 seconds cued by the sound of the chimes or piano	Noticing feelings of connection in mind, body and breath through the experience of mindful movement	Modified yoga nidra using the visualization of shining stars all over the body	Coherent Breathing using the audio track. Feeling connected through breath	Do you feel more connection to yourself? To others? To your world?

TECHNICAL NOTES ON EACH PRACTICE

Psycho-education sets the theme for the week, which is threaded through every practice. It introduces the breathing practice and any new techniques.

Initial centring and breathing – clearing space in the mind, promoting body and breath awareness, practising breathing technique.

Simple arm movement to connect breath with movement and release shoulders.

Raising and lowering arms – further breath and movement (eventually breath-led movement) and turning the palms to reflect transitions (later, pauses) between inhale and exhale.

Shoulder mobilization of the shoulder girdle, and then girdle and glenohumeral joint, with side bend to lengthen fascia and promote freedom of movement in the chest.

Simple neck stretch involving flexion and optional rotation to release neck muscles and counteract common patterns of hyperextension in the cervical spine, which inhibit breathing, affect posture and can increase sympathetic drive.

Initial twist in a chair to begin spinal mobilization. Contrary twist to maximize mobilization.

Initial backbend to connect to thoracic spine – the focus of all backbending in the protocol.

Transition to re-centre if moving from chair to mat.

Activation of deep core muscles, transversus abdominus, internal obliques and thoracolumbar fascia for spinal support.

Extending the breath, shoulder opener and gentle backbend with awareness to avoiding lumbar arching by exhaling navel to spine. Continuation of core awakening.

Release for lower back and sacroiliac joint.

Ankle mobilization, hip opening and (with straight leg) hip flexor lengthening. Double legs to chest to release lower back further.

Further abdominal strength using deep and superficial muscles, and strengthening pelvic floor.

Hip opening – particularly effective in the supine position without weight going into the joints.

Tense-relax practice to highlight sensations of tension and relaxation to develop patient skills and proprioception. Becoming aware of tension and being able to switch it off. Held version magnifies contrast between tense-release phases.

Dynamic supine twist with shoulders and head in opposite directions maximizes spinal mobilization. Mat version has advantage of taking the spine out of gravity and therefore out of compression of inter-vertebral discs.

Held twist to go deeper.

Cross-crawl aids horizontal integration of right and left hemispheres of the brain. Supports overall coordination, stretches hamstrings and releases shoulders.

Pelvic tilts release sacroiliac joint and bring awareness to core muscles supporting the correct pelvic position in the following backbend to avoid over-working lumbar area.

Dynamic bridge opens spine and mobilizes on exhale phase. Less effective in a chair due to gravitational compression on inter vertebral discs.

Held bridge supports further thoracic mobility and core and leg strength. Thoracic opening only in chair version.

Dynamic hamstring stretching with knee bending on each inhale to avoid over-stimulation of the stretch reflex arc. Held stretch develops further flexibility in these muscles, which when short correlate with poor posture and lower back pain.

Thread the needle develops further hip opening. A cautious approach is taken, as the pose uses the leg as a lever to open the hip. The knee is vulnerable, hence the dorsiflexion of the ankle to activate supporting muscles around the knee joint.

Cat pose as included mobilizes over 70 spinal joints with each movement. Knees padded for all students (not just those with knee problems) in recognition of poor design of knees for any weight-bearing. Hands placed in front of shoulders to avoid 90-degree angle on wrists, which is beyond normal range of movement. Chair versions to minimize weight into the wrists and shoulders for patients with problems in these areas.

Easy sphinx to approach backbending in an inclusive way. Opportunity to ensure patients understand the importance of keeping the front of the pelvis pressing down into the mat to avoid lower back strain. The chair version is dynamic because holding arm position would be too tiring. Supported chair version offered.

Lifting and lowering the spine out of gravity is a safe way to build back strength and prevents future back problems. It strengthens the erector spinae muscles, among others. The chair version has the same benefit. Kneeling and a chair can be used for a more horizontal spine.

Single leg raises strengthen the gluteus maximus and medius, and some lower back muscles. Weak glutes are common and correlate with lower back pain. The chair version does not achieve the same result; supported kneeling with a chair does.

Dynamic downward facing dog builds arm and shoulder strength, and supports core engagement and spinal lengthening. The dynamic version is more inclusive for those with medicated and controlled elevated blood pressure who have been told they can do mild short-hold inversions. The chair or back-of-chair versions avoid any head-below-heart movement and are safe for many cardiovascular patients.

Held downward facing dog builds further strength. Options to avoid inversion.

Transition to standing, with shoulder, wrist and hand mobilization to counterpose weight-bearing work just completed. The chair version provides the same mobilization benefits.

Breath and movement with sweeping arms connects patients to a fuller breath, releases the shoulders and awakens the feet by toe and heel lifting. Preparation for standing work and balances.

Sun salutations – inclusive design of this version allows mat- and chair-based students to work simultaneously through a 14-breath sequence that stretches the whole body and supports cardiovascular, respiratory and lymphatic health. Includes lengthening of the back line, back strengthening, side stretching and shoulder release.

Dynamic warrior 1 stretches the hip flexors, calves and Achilles, while opening the chest in a meditative flowing and breath-led movement. Correct alignment needed, with feet hip width apart and back foot only turned out slightly. The chair version works well, or support from the back of the chair.

Dynamic warrior 2 opens one hip at a time, stretches the adductors and works the foot muscles. Upper body coordination with the lower body creates another meditative and flowing movement led by the breath. The chair version works well, or support from the back of the chair.

Inclusive heron balance allows patients to gain confidence in balance. Early weeks allow only the arm movement and weight shift between the feet before alternate heels are lifted and then the whole leg. Raising and lowering the leg with the breath may be as far as some patients progress, as held balances are difficult and can be demoralizing. A chair or wall is used for support where needed. All patients who can stand are encouraged to do the balance work because of the high rates of hospitalization due to falls, particularly among elderly people.

Tree pose is more advanced and may be unsuitable for those with hip or knee problems. It can be taught dynamically or statically with a range of inclusive foot and arm positions.

Inversion – the legs-on-chair version is encouraged for most patients.

Relaxation – comfort is the watchword here. A range of options are offered.

Final breathing practice can be done sitting on the mat or back in the chair. All patients come back to the chair after this practice for group discussion.

CHAPTER 6

Learning to Relax

Everything is impermanent. Knowing this, just relax.

Ancient saying

Relaxation is vital to health; it gives our minds and bodies time to build resources and restore wear and tear arising from daily life processes and unexpected stress. The ability to relax is not a given, and often people need to cultivate the practice of relaxation. The yoga method focuses on the importance of relaxation, by ending each class with a resting pose. This time of nourishment and self-care helps us to enter a more settled state of body and mind in which we are more likely to experience what we might describe as our authentic Self.

WHAT IS RELAXATION?
The answer to this question is highly individual. Some may say they relax with a glass of wine on a Friday evening and watch a movie; others may attend a live sporting event and enter a high state of arousal through shouting, chanting and singing – but still call it relaxation. Some relax by taking recreational drugs – or enjoy the simple legal "buzz" of a flat white or a few beers with friends.

The *Oxford English Dictionary* reflects these different aspects of relaxation:

A state of being free from tension and anxiety.
Recreation or rest, especially after a period of work.
The loss of tension in a part of the body, especially in a muscle when it ceases to contract.

In yoga, relaxation is a state of calm mind, in which the constant dis-cursive thoughts momentarily reduce their intensity or entirely cease. As this goes against the grain of how many of us think, we could say relaxation is active; it requires mental training and effort.

YIHA's understanding of what constitutes relaxation in a mind-body practice like yoga is informed by Dr Herbert Benson, professor, author and cardiologist, and a founder of Harvard's Benson-Henry Institute, a mind-body research institute. His book *The Relaxation Response* was the first to set out the scientific underpinning for the physiological processes that inspire relaxation (the movement from sympathetic drive to para-sympathetic response). He named the state of deep rest he discovered the relaxation response. This state is one in which cells significantly reduce their metabolic rate, providing an opportunity for cellular res-toration. Cellular metabolism includes the catalysing of energy for life processes and in of itself requires lots of energy. Reducing the metabolic rate allows us to rest at the core of our being (Benson, 2007). Dr Benson's studies in the 1960s and 1970s revealed that entering the relaxation response brings marked positive changes at systems and cellular levels. Recent research even demonstrates that entering the physiological state of the relaxation response gives rise to positive changes in genetic expression (Saatcioglu, 2013).

Dr Benson's approach to achieving the relaxation response involves the following steps (Benson, 2016).

- Repeat a movement, word or sound.

- Disregard intrusive thoughts that arise in the mind.

Benson says these first two steps break the chain of everyday thinking.

- Breathe slowly, and on the exhale say your word, phrase or prayer. (During Yoga4Health relaxations, patients are invited to repeat phrases like "Exhale down to the ground".)

- Do this practice for at least 5 minutes, while continuing to disre-gard the thoughts that will inevitably intrude into the mind (with a relaxed "Oh well" and return to the chosen word, phrase or prayer).

He recommends this as a daily practice lasting, ideally, 10–15 minutes and says "You are tapping into a resource that is within yourself that is opposite to stress" (Benson, 2007).

Regular relaxation practice can lead to:

- reduced heart rate

- slower and deeper breathing

- lower blood pressure

- reduced muscular tension

- changes in genetic expression that help to reduce inflammation.

At the end of every session in the ten-week programme, Yoga4Health patients are led through a relaxation practice aligned with the class theme. Patients are privy to a broad experience of different relaxation techniques. These relaxations are also made available as MP3 files, kindly recorded for us by Yoga4Health teacher Leanne Antonia. In their own practice and after the course has ended, patients can experiment with the different relaxations and use the ones that work best for them. Or they may use the relaxation practices as a launch pad to further their own journey into yoga and relaxation.

During our evaluation of the effectiveness of the Yoga4Health programme, many patients have told us how much they have benefited from the relaxation. Some have described it as a rare time in their week when they completely switch off; others have said that they experience improved sleep during the night after their weekly class. We think this is not merely due to the relaxation itself, but also to situating the relaxation after gentle stretching, when tension melts away and the body is primed to enter a state of deep rest.

THE SCIENCE BEHIND RELAXATION

Most people can benefit from relaxation, including those referred to the programme with stress or mild to moderate anxiety/depression; they all benefit from relaxation. However, people with severe anxiety and deeper depressive states (who would fall into our exclusionary criteria) may not be able to close their eyes and go inward without being lost in rumination. As a result, the type of relaxation practice offered in this course might make them feel worse.

It is for these reasons that most of the research on relaxation has focused on using techniques to address less acute mental health problems, including stress and mild depression.

Yoga classes make use of the inclusion of physical activity through the *asana* practice before relaxation to help students/patients work through layers of stress. This prepares the ground for a more effective relaxation.

A study carried out in Australia gave two groups of students a tenweek course of either yoga or relaxation. This randomized control trial involved 131 people from South Australia who had mild to moderate levels of stress. The researchers found that yoga was as effective as relaxation at reducing stress and anxiety and at improving health. Yoga was additionally found to be more effective than relaxation at improving mental health (Smith *et al.*, 2007). By combining yoga with formal relaxation, we get both benefits together, hopefully heightening the overall effect on wellbeing!

In the UK, the NHS recommends relaxation techniques, including reducing muscle tension and calming the mind, to help patients manage feelings of anxiety and learn to control them.

RETURNING TO BALANCE

Yoga relaxation techniques aim to restore physical and mental balance to promote optimum health. Scientists use the medical term "homeostasis" to define physiological balance in the body. As mentioned earlier, a main cause of imbalance is when the two aspects of the ANS (sympathetic and parasympathetic) become dysregulated with hyperactivity of the sympathetic system. Groundbreaking insight into this area was provided by Professor of Psychiatry at the University of North Carolina and Distinguished Scientist at the Kinsey Institute, Stephen Porges, when he published his now widely disseminated polyvagal theory (Porges, 2001). Polyvagal theory has revolutionized the understanding of autonomic physiology and what it means to be in a physiologically relaxed state by setting out the neurophysiological foundations of emotions, attachment, communication and self-regulation. The theory expresses why in any given social situation, some people may feel relaxed and happy while others may feel uncertainty, fear and a lack of safety or even a total sense of frozenness accompanied by an inability to connect.

Optimal neurological and systems functioning necessitates that we feel safe. Achieving this state involves us reading hundreds of social cues, such as facial expressions, voice tone and gestures through the vista of our own personal association with these inputs, coupled with certain biological inherent imperatives. For example, a melodious voice and gentle gaze is likely to afford a sense of ease. These enable the mind to shape our feelings and experience of social situations.

Polyvagal theory postulates that our "social engagement system" evolved to enable us to create and recreate tribal bonds and social connection during human evolution. If our "neuroception", as Porges calls it, perceives a threat, it will adjust autonomic activity so that we may respond aptly to this threat in order to survive.

Polyvagal theory describes three primary subdivisions of the ANS, which evolved over time. Two of these divisions are mediated by the vagal system, hence the term "polyvagal theory". Each system promotes survival in its own way. The phylogenetically oldest (oldest within the evolutionary record) is the "dorsal vagal circuit", a part of the nervous system that enables us to shut down or "freeze" when a situation is neurologically perceived as life-threatening. Freeze promotes survival as predators tend to respond more to motion. In the human context, freeze may also prevent a violent attack from becoming more intense. If this strategy worked during a highly traumatic situation, the nervous system may call on it during reminders of the event, even without an imminent threat. The next is the SNS, known as the fight-or-flight system. This helps us to flee or fight when facing a perceived threat. The division is purported by Porges to be unique to mammals and is known as the ventral vagus circuit. This circuit promotes survival through bonding, where others help us to regulate our nervous system through safe interactions, hold us when we are sad, tend to us when we are ill and support us when there is threat. This is the circuit associated with the social engagement network. The complex neural pathways of this system not only influence and affect heart rate and breathing, but also influence our ability to listen, movement of facial muscles and voice modulation. Additionally, ventral vagal activity is associated with reduced use of resources of the body and promotes greater health. One can increase the activity of this system through practices that enhance parasympathetic drive.

This pioneering theory not only helps us understand what is

necessary for a truly physiologically relaxed state, but has also transformed understanding of mental health. In addition to the above, Porges has explained that 80% of the fibres of the ventral vagus nerve move from body to brain, suggesting the body has a superior role in regulating emotion (Porges, 2017). This highlights the essential nature of body-based therapy, influencing psychiatry, nursing, mind-body work, yoga therapy, trauma recovery, parenting and education – to name but a few – and, of course, yoga teaching. Yoga teachers wishing to have relaxed and happy students can usefully grasp the essential elements of the theory to take steps to ensure that students/patients have the best chance of the vagal response that supports connection, safety and a deep sense of belonging and ease. This includes things like an elongated exhale, which activates the ventral vagus network, delivering the relaxation activities with a melodious voice and holding the discussion with kindness and clear social skills. At YIHA, we believe that polyvagal theory actually provides further evidence to support social prescribing. The forging of bonds, thus activating the ventral vagal circuit, is healthy for the body. Polyvagal theory also highlights the importance of kindness and care in any social-prescribing programme. Finally, as practices like yoga increase the activity of the polyvagal circuit, YIHA believes that yoga may be one of the most useful social-prescription options.

Creation of safe space and nurturing social connection on the Yoga-4Health protocol is a prerequisite for the effectiveness of the postures, breathing practices and concentration that lead the student towards mental and physical balance. This state of mind is then deepened during the relaxation offered near the end of class.

In B. K. S. Iyengar's classic book *Light on Yoga*, the relaxation pose *savasana* (corpse pose) is described as "one of the most difficult to master" because it is much harder to keep the mind still when the body is not moving (1965, p.422).

Experienced yoga practitioners with a steadier mind may find the process of relaxation relatively easy. They may attend classes in which relaxation can last for 30 minutes or more and where there are sustained periods of silence. For patients and others with a less-developed yoga practice, it is important to offer a guided relaxation practice of 10–15 minutes (this is even shorter in Week 1), avoiding long periods of silence that might lead to mind wandering.

The ten relaxations offered on the programme progress in the following way.

- Week 1 – A brief period of tensing and releasing different parts of the body, followed by breathing in and out of different parts of the body, while rotating awareness around the body from the feet to the head.

- Week 2 – A brief period of tensing and releasing different parts of the body, followed by relaxing while focusing on the points of contact between the body and the ground. Awareness is again taken from one part of the body to another, starting at the feet.

- Week 3 – A brief period of tensing and releasing different parts of the body, followed by developing the sense of contact to the ground, in line with the grounding theme of Weeks 2–4. Using a lengthened exhale while visualizing different parts of the body and imagining those areas releasing more deeply to the ground.

- Week 4 – Similar to Week 3, but with the addition of a lengthened "ocean breath" on inhale as well as exhaling down to the ground.

- Week 5 – Rotation of awareness around the body, with a focus on experiencing space in each part of the body, in line with the theme of spaciousness.

- Week 6 – Rotation of awareness around the body, with a focus on experiencing space in each part of the body, in line with the theme of spaciousness (same as Week 5).

- Week 7 – Rotation of awareness around the body, with the patients invited to notice every sensation they feel in each area. Links to theme of awareness to bodily sensations.

- Week 8 – Awareness is moved from side to side in the body to link to the theme of balance. The sensations on one side of the body are compared with those on the other to develop proprioception.

- Week 9 – The theme of change is explored by noticing the small shifts in sensations. How they rise and fall away, become more intense or dissipate. This builds further refined awareness of sensation in the body and teaches the impermanence of what we may be feeling at any given moment.

- Week 10 – Connection is the theme for the final week of the course, and this relaxation offers a rather different experience of a modified yoga nidra. Yoga nidra means "yogic sleep" and is a deeper state of relaxation in which objects being visualized (or imagined) by the patient help them to transcend the physical body. In this case, patients imagine placing shining stars all over their body, until their body transforms into a body of light. This relaxation links to the yogic idea of promoting the free flow of *prana* (subtle energy) around the energy body, the *pranamaya kosha*, while also giving people a feeling of deep connection to the universe. The Week 10 relaxation ends with patients counting their breaths backwards from 20 to 1 and then enjoying a short period of stillness and silence.

Relaxation scripts are provided to all our Yoga4Health teachers, although they are not expected to deliver the scripts in their exact form. There is leeway to adapt language and pace and to reinterpret the theme of the relaxation to meet the needs of their cohort of patients and their own teaching style.

You can enjoy all ten Yoga4Health relaxations by downloading them as MP3 files from the YIHA website.[1]

REFERENCES

Benson, H. (2007). *The Relaxation Response.* New York: William Morrow & Co.
Benson, H. (2016). *Relaxation Response: Dr. Herbert Benson Teaches You the Basics.* Accessed on 15/10/2021 at: www.youtube.com/watch?v=nBcsFuoFRp8.
Iyengar, B. K. S. (1965). *Light on Yoga.* New York: Schocken Books.
Porges, S. (2001). 'The polyvagal theory: Phylogenetic substrates of a social nervous system.' *International Journal of Psychophysiology 42*, 123–146.
Porges, S. W. (2017). *The Pocket Guide to The Polyvagal Theory.* New York: W. W. Norton & Co.
Saatcioglu, F. (2013). 'Regulation of gene expression by yoga, meditation and related practices: A review of recent studies.' *Asian Journal of Psychiatry 6*, 1, 74–77.
Smith, C., Hancock, H., Blake-Mortimer, J. and Eckert, K. (2007). 'A randomised comparative trial of yoga and relaxation to reduce stress and anxiety.' *Complementary Therapies in Medicine 15*, 2, 77–83.

---

1   www.yogainhealthcarealliance.com/resources

CHAPTER 7

Reflective Practice
and Learning

*By three methods we may learn wisdom. First by reflection,
which is the noblest; second, by imitation, which is the easiest;
and third, by experience, which is the most bitter.*

Confucius

The yoga tradition consistently teaches the importance of exploration of the inner world. Contemplation can be honed through *asana*, as the yogi focuses his or her mind on sensations arising in the body while moving through their practice. As yoga naturally involves mindful attention to the self, practitioners notice their own reactions to poses, and those of others in the class, guided by the teacher. This can stimulate a reappraisal of responses, setting the groundwork for transformation. This process is further defined via breath practices and finally through meditation, in which the mind looks inward at itself. For people attending a weekly yoga class, the self-reflection that results from turning attention inwards instead of outwards for the duration of the class promotes awareness and mindfulness.

Transforming behaviour through self-reflection is a process embraced in thousands of self-help books and psychological therapies. It is also rooted in yoga's *yamas* (duty, restraint, outward observances) and *niyamas* (ways of living, inner observances) set out in Patanjali's *Yoga Sutras*.

YAMAS – OUTER OBSERVANCES FOR OUR INTERACTIONS WITH OTHER PEOPLE AND THE WORLD

- *Ahimsa* – nonviolence

- *Satya* – truthfulness

- *Asteya* – non-stealing

- *Brahmacharya* – avoiding excess/conserving vital energy

- *Aparigraha* – non-possessiveness, non-greed

NIYAMAS – WAYS OF LIVING

- *Saucha* – purity of body and mind

- *Santosha* – contentment

- *Tapas* – effort and self-discipline

- *Svadhyaya* – self-study and inner exploration

- *Ishvara pranidhana* – surrender to a higher purpose/consciousness

The benefits of everyday reflection have found their way into contemporary theories and approaches to education because they make learning more effective. Pioneers in this field include Schon (1991), who developed the concept of "reflection-in-action", and Kolb, who wrote about the "experiential learning cycle" (Leeds Safeguarding Children Partnership, n.d.). Both were attempting to bridge the gap between what we think is happening (often at a superficial level) and what is actually happening.

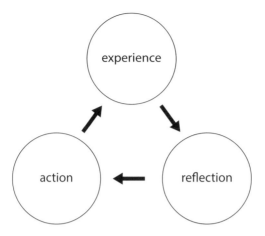

Jasper's Reflective Cycle

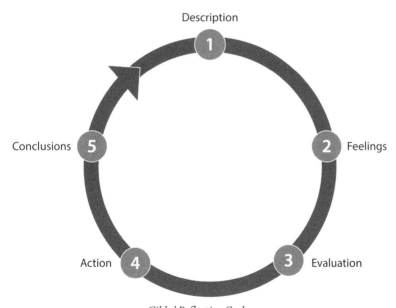

Gibbs' Reflective Cycle

There are a number of theoretical models of reflective practice. In Jasper's reflective cycle (Jasper, 2003), we see a simple process that anyone could follow: experience, leading to reflection, leading to refined action in the future. Other educational models, like Gibbs' reflective cycle (The University of Edinburgh, 2020), include additional steps in the reflective practice cycle. Both have the common purpose of making a person's learning deeper and more meaningful through a feedback loop of reflective practice. Luigiani Mortari describes reflection as fundamental to thinking:

> Learning the practice of reflection is fundamental because it allows people to engage into a thoughtful relationship with the world-life and thus gain an awake stance about one's lived experience. Reflection is a crucial cognitive practice... (Mortari, 2015, p.1177)

Reflective practice has been shown to improve emotional intelligence and a more positive sense of Self. Leading yoga therapist Marlysa Sullivan considers the *yamas* and *niyamas* as essential ingredients in the healing power of yoga, as she claims they shift perspective on pain in exchange for virtue, self-inquiry and a life led with meaning (Sullivan, 2018). Although these values seems to arise organically through the practice of yoga, a wise teacher will thread these through class either covertly or overtly in a manner that supports student transformation.

For students, guided reflective practice is a tool to deepen understanding of experience in class and can seep into the ability to reflect in everyday life. This reflection helps us to evolve strategies to deal with situations more skilfully from a place of wisdom and grounding.

Let's consider an adverse event, such as getting into an argument with a colleague. You feel strongly that a particular course of action is required; they feel equally strongly that a different process should be followed. Tempers flare and the heated argument results in both parties feeling hurt and unheard. Reflection after the event might mean you acknowledge that both courses of action lead to the same destination. You disagree on the detail of how to get there but share a common goal. Perhaps you can see how both approaches can be integrated. Perhaps you also reflect that you did not listen as attentively as you could have and were too focused on putting your own views forwards; you had already made up your mind. Perhaps you may even imagine why the other person was so attached to their perspective and understand where their entrenched view may be arising from, in the same way that your entrenched view has roots somewhere. You may further reflect that moving together as a team and maintaining cohesion and shared goals is more important than getting everything that you want. Armed with this knowledge and increased self-awareness, you begin afresh the next day, apologizing to your colleague for losing your temper and asking if you might both reconsider what should be done in a way that leaves both of you feeling valued and heard.

Such a course of action is more likely to lead to a positive resolution of the problem and avoid blame and recriminations that might otherwise pollute the working relationship. The causes of the negative interaction will have been tackled and replaced with a positive action that transcends what went before and heals wounds. A process of more skilful action following reflection.

The Viniyoga teacher Paul Harvey describes yoga as "skilful living". Through practice, expanded awareness and the ongoing study of yoga texts, like Patanjali's *Yoga Sutras*, we become better equipped to operate in the world with more happiness, equanimity and poise (Harvey, 2021). Alyson Ross, in her 2013 qualitative analysis (a study looking at arising themes in research), found that those who practised yoga reported it improved relationships with others. In fact, she called her research paper "I am a nice person when I do yoga!!!" (Ross, 2014).

REFLECTIVE PRACTICE IN THE YOGA4HEALTH PROGRAMME

Reflection is different from spoon-feeding someone information; reflection calls on the person to investigate for themselves. It highlights self-developed knowledge and empowers people to be creators of their own destiny. As yoga professionals, we hold a fine balance between offering directives that support patients in moving from one staging post to the next and cuing self-led investigation, leading to a myriad of possible answers to their questions of self-enquiry.

During every Yoga4Health session, the teacher integrates the weekly theme into class by regularly inviting students to notice how they feel, what they feel and where they feel it. Often, open-ended questions are used. How is your breath in this pose? How does your connection to the ground feel? How does the intention to find space in the body affect the mind? If you are struggling with the balance this week, how does that make you feel? It is not the teacher's job to define experiences, just to invite the self-enquiry among students that will deepen their understanding of themselves and their experience of the yoga practices they are doing.

By hearing the teacher mention a range of possible experiences, such as discomfort or comfort in a forward bend (depending on hamstring length), students are also drawn into an attitude of self-enquiry that is without judgement and designed to encourage kindness towards themselves and others. They learn that their experience will not be the same as anyone else's experience. Everyone in the class is having a different experience of the same practice.

At the end of class, patients are given the opportunity to express their reflections during the group discussion. This builds on the reflection-in-action they will have done during the class.

To support reflection outside of class, students are given a list of questions in the manual to help them contemplate their own lives and how the practice is influencing their experience. Notably, the students are regularly asked if there are known impediments to home practice and how these might be overcome.

SHARED DECISION-MAKING AND CO-CREATION

Two further ideas that are becoming embedded in primary care in the UK and relate to reflective practice are shared decision-making (briefly mentioned earlier) and co-creation. We have seen that the medium through which information is imparted can invite passivity or self-efficacy. NHS England's current ten-year plan for the NHS envisages universal personalised care, which puts the patient at the centre of their treatment and health. Doctors are being retrained to conduct consultations in a way that leads to shared decision-making about whatever drugs or treatment might be suitable for their patient's health condition. Previously, doctors might have assumed they were the experts and simply informed patients about what they need; doctor knows best. This has been replaced by a shared decision-making model in which the patient ultimately decides they want a particular treatment.

This can be seen as co-creating the next step in that patient's healthcare. Co-creation is a central idea in social prescribing when describing the relationship between a patient/client and the Social Prescribing Link Worker. Conversations and discussions will invite the client to reflect on a range of options that might meet their needs and then settle on an agreed way forwards with their Link Worker.

We infuse co-creation into the Yoga4Health programme right from the start when we begin initial contact with the patients and find out their needs. The discussion is open and promotes dialogue and self-efficacy. If the patient arrives at the belief that this is the programme that will help them with their problems, we achieve more commitment than if they simply meet the referral criteria and are "allowed" on the programme.

LEARNING STYLES

Everyone tends to have a preferred way of learning. One person may thrive from hearing instructions. Another may prefer to see what it is they are meant to do. A third will only really understand when they do it themselves. Most people can receive information in all three learning styles but find sessions more effective when their preferred learning style is included.

In a yoga class, the teacher demonstrates practices (visual), gives simple clear instructions to enter and leave a practice (auditory) and enables students to have their own experience of the practice (kinaesthetic). This creates a rich learning environment and raises the chances that students will understand and reflect.

Yoga4Health teachers provide access to home-practice videos for those who like to see what to do, audio tracks of those practices for those happier hearing what to do and relentless encouragement to undertake home practice for those who learn best by just doing.

Additional resources in the form of handouts and links to articles and videos in the emails we send every week to patients are an additional support to learning. One handout that might be given is Maslow's hierarchy of needs, which helps patients consider their own needs and what is necessary to achieve them while undertaking the ten-week programme.

MASLOW'S HIERARCHY OF NEEDS AND THE YOGA4HEALTH PROGRAMME

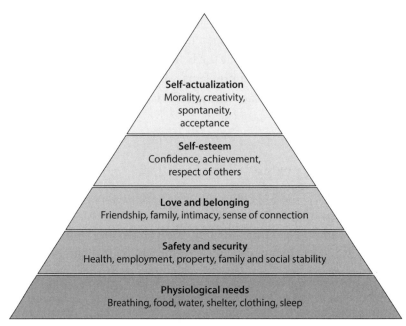

Maslow's Hierarchy of Needs

The psychologist Abraham Maslow first came up with his Theory of Human Motivation in 1943 (50minutes.com, 2015). He recognized that basic needs in the lowest two levels of the triangle need to be met before any higher needs can be aspired to. A person must have food, water, clothing and shelter to survive, and feel enough safety and security from things like family and social connection to have enough personal resources and resilience to make progress.

As we move up to love and belonging, we begin to see that the friendships and social connection support this tier. Via relationships built on the Yoga4Health programme, we hope to galvanize this level of need and prop up others. Self-esteem, also in Maslow's model, is a critical element of the programme, empowering patients through an appropriate yoga practice in an inclusive and non-competitive environment. How the teacher relates to patients, holds the space and encourages respect within the group via ground rules and discussion reinforces this layer of Maslow's hierarchy.

It is only when all the underlying tiers are in place that people can find themselves in a position to explore and "actualize" the highest needs of morality, spontaneity, creativity and acceptance.

THE VOCABULARY OF TEACHING

Reflection also helps YIHA to improve its programme. For example, through discussion with its teaching community, YIHA has refined its language. We understand that language is a primary vehicle of reflection and so it must be carefully considered, especially as inclusivity is a major tenet of the programme.

This is easier said than done, because there are so many hidden barriers to full inclusion. "OK guys, now we are going to..." is a common start to a sentence used by female yoga teachers leading a class of mainly women. Why guys? We have made a lot of strides in eradicating overt sexism, but in our use of language there are still phrases that hark back to a patriarchal society. Reflection on the language we use is important. Our vocabulary of teaching must continue to evolve and not be stuck in the past.

Our teachers aim to use language that is secular and non-discriminatory. They strive to create a neutral space in which everyone feels accepted and can be themselves. At the same time, we acknowledge that our world view is shaped by our own cultural and life experiences. We should be prepared to learn and reflect without judgement. The new language around gender and sexuality is an example of how the landscape of inclusion is not static, and everyone holding space for others must keep up with developments.

Within each cohort of patients, there is likely to be a wide range of views, and sometimes this can include prejudices. The teacher's space-holding and ability to reflect on the needs of the group must be strong enough to uphold safety and define clearly what is not acceptable language or behaviour whenever it arises.

SAFEGUARDING

Maintaining safety in class includes having enough knowledge and training to ensure adult safeguarding. All Yoga4Health teachers are required to hold an up-to-date training in this area so that they can protect vulnerable adults, spot the signs of abuse and know the correct procedures to follow when a safeguarding concern arises. We regularly hold online training and policy update sessions for our teachers and have a suite of PCI-approved policies that are reviewed and updated regularly and include:

- safeguarding

- code of conduct

- malpractice

- health and safety

- complaints

- equality, diversity and inclusion

- bullying and harassment

- privacy.

The professional context that Yoga4Health teachers operate in is described in the *Core Values of Personalised Care*, which is included in our PCI-approved training programme (Personalised Care Institute, 2021).

REFERENCES

50minutes.com (2015). *Maslow's Hierarchy of Needs*. Accessed on 15/10/2021 at: www.50minutes.com/title/maslows-hierarchy-of-needs.

Harvey, P. (2021). *Yoga Studies*. Accessed on 16/9/2021 at: https://yogastudies.org.

Jasper, M. (2003). *Beginning Reflective Practice*. Cheltenham: Nelson Thornes.

Leeds Safeguarding Children Partnership (n.d.). *Kolb's Cycle of Reflective Practice*. Accessed on 10/01/2022 at: https://www.leedsscp.org.uk/practitioners/working-with-families/practitioners-toolkit/kolbs-cycle.

Mortari, L. (2015). 'Reflectivity in research practice: An overview of different perspectives.' *International Journal of Qualitative Methods*. December 2015. doi: 10.1177/1609406915618045.

Personalised Care Institute (2021). *Curriculum*. Accessed on 16/9/2021 at: www.personalisedcareinstitute.org.uk/wp-content/uploads/2021/06/The-personalised-care-curriculum.pdf.

Ross, A. (2014). '"I am a nice person when I do yoga!!!" A qualitative analysis of how yoga affects relationships.' *Journal of Holistic Nursing 32*, 2, 67–77.

Schon, D. A. (1991). *The Reflective Practitioner: How Professionals Think in Action*. Abingdon-on-Thames, Oxfordshire: Routledge.

Sullivan, M. B. (2018). *Understanding Yoga Therapy: Applied Philosophy and Science for Health and Well-Being*. New York: Routledge.

The University of Edinburgh (2020). *Gibbs' Reflective Cycle*. Accessed on 15/10/2021 at: www.ed.ac.uk/reflection/reflectors-toolkit/reflecting-on-experience/gibbs-reflective-cycle.

CHAPTER 8

Your Lifelong Journey in Health and Happiness

*Happiness and freedom begin with a clear understanding of one
principle. Some things are within your control. And some things are not.*

Epictetus, Greek Stoic philosopher

The Yoga4Health ten-week programme aims to bring about positive
lifestyle change in patients who are at risk of becoming chronically ill.
The intensity of ten consecutive weeks of two-hour sessions, which is
backed up by daily home practice and psycho-education themes, including those on mindfulness, diet and exercise, plays a part in supporting
this positive change.

As we saw in Chapter 2, the results from the University of Westminster evaluation of Yoga4Health revealed that three months after
the ten-week programme ended, patients were still practising yoga, on
average, just over two days a week. Some 44% had begun attending a
local class, and half were continuing to use the home-practice resources
online or in their patient manuals. This is a high level of patient activation and suggests that the ten-week programme has a long-term impact
on health and lifestyle choices.

However, lifestyle change is difficult. Our minds are very adept at
justifying the current choices we make. Another bottle of wine gets
opened; an extra unnecessary helping of pudding is consumed; the
gym membership taken out in early January turns out to be one of our
most expensive and unnecessary purchases because we are attending so

infrequently. We often know that we need to adopt a different lifestyle but delay making changes.

This point is not made to induce guilt or shame, not least because such feelings are an ineffective mechanism to motivate change. Rather, it is to acknowledge that this is a common experience for all of us. The solution offered by yoga is to understand the nature of the mind and, in a step-by-step manner, learn to exercise a measure of control over it. Not in a regimented sense but in a kind and compassionate way. The uncontrolled mind can be likened to a toddler whose attention is grabbed by whatever the senses perceive. A toy, a cake – they feel intensely that they must have it NOW! Adults may not throw a tantrum when their desires are unfulfilled (although some do!) but may instead feel unhappy, worried and restless.

THE MIND

The journey towards a steadier mind is the path of yoga. Only by bringing the mind to a place of peace and insight can true joy and ease arise. The *Katha Upanishad* conveys its wisdom through an imagined conversation between a spiritual seeker, Naciketas, and the Lord of Death. The Lord of Death says a person is like a chariot drawn by horses. The true Self is a passenger, the chariot the body, the intellect the charioteer and the mind the reins. The senses are represented by the horses, and the sensory objects all around are the many paths that the horses could gallop along.

> When a person lacks understanding, and the mind is never controlled
> The senses do not obey him/her, as bad horses...
> But when a person has understanding, and the mind is ever controlled
> The senses do obey him/her, as good horses... (*Katha Upanishad*, chapter 3, verses 5–6; Olivelle, 2008)

Lord Krishna has a similar message for his charioteer disciple, Arjuna, in the *Bhagavad Gita*:

> The illumined One has learned to deftly withdraw the senses from the attractions of the world, just as a tortoise naturally pulls in its limbs to protect itself...

Much of one's spiritual discipline must therefore focus on taming wayward senses and being ever vigilant against the treacherousness of the senses.

The refinement of an individual or a society is measured by the yardstick of how well greed and desires are controlled. (*Bhagavad Gita*, chapter 2, verses 58 and 60; Hawley, 2012)

According to Patanjali, the vacillating waves of perception entering the mind through the senses should be stilled by consistent earnest practice and dispassionate non-attachment.

Non-attachment is the mastery of consciousness,
wherein one is free from craving objects of enjoyment,
whether they have been perceived or imagined... (*Yoga Sutras of Patanjali*, chapter 1, verse 15; Stiles, 2001)

We can summarize these teachings as: the senses are powerful drivers of desires in the mind and it might not be a good idea to follow them on their never-ending meandering journey. If we want to feel in control of our lives and have a sense of who we really are, we must cultivate the mind.

There is another concept to add here so that we have a more complete picture of how control of the senses fits into lifestyle change and a life rooted in yoga practice. Yoga suggests that there are two aspects to mind: lower mind, *manas*, and higher mind, *buddhi*, or intellect. It is the lower mind of *manas* that craves sensory input from the eyes (sight), nose (smell), ears (sound), tongue (taste) and skin (touch) and also gives rise to a host of perceptions in conjunction with the senses. You walk past the cake shop and see the iced bun, you smell the delicious aroma of freshly baked bread, your taste buds tingle as you salivate and you experience a strong desire to walk in, buy the iced bun and enjoy it. Then you look at your watch and realize it is only 9.30am. You just had breakfast. You are not really hungry. You are trying to lose weight and get fit. Is that iced bun really going to help? This is your *buddhi*, your intellect, bringing discriminative analysis to the desire and enabling you to step back from it and assess its worth.

However, let's not be too strict about all this. You might equally look at your watch and think you don't really need that right now. But buying one and sharing it with your partner at afternoon tea might be a nice treat and still within your regime of controlling your diet. Still, this might be the mind playing tricks on us, allowing us what we desire and providing a more palatable scenario to fulfil it. *Manas* is tricky!

The teachings of yoga provide practical advice on living in ways that allow us to be in control of our senses, rather than our senses being in control of us. The yogic advice is that following the senses can only lead to temporary pleasure before slipping back into suffering. Those senses can never be fully satisfied, only temporarily sated. After that, new desires will arise that destroy equanimity and put us right back on the carousel – going round and round, chasing never-ending desires.

Cultivating the habit of non-attachment is fundamental to getting off the merry-go-round. This entails creating enough space in the mind to intercept desires and emotions before we have activated habitual patterns of thinking and behaving in response to them. Sometimes this habit is described as cultivating the witness, and it relates to the idea that we are not our thoughts but an enduring presence of Self that lies beneath.

Cultivating this witness is an aspect of reflection discussed in Chapter 7. If someone makes you angry, you notice that you are becoming angry. You treat yourself kindly and wonder why you are feeling this way. Is it necessary or justifiable to become angry, or are you responding out of habit? Can you show empathy towards the other person and understand what they are dealing with that might explain their behaviour towards you?

Over time, this attitude of non-attachment and self-enquiry creates more and more space in the mind until your default position becomes listening, watchfulness and curiosity – followed by a considered response to whatever is going on. You are not going to get it right every time, and you may still get angry and unreasonable yourself. We are not perfect. But you have moved from a place of knee-jerk to heightened awareness and mindfulness.

Couples wishing to adopt a looked-after child in the UK undergo up to two years of training in therapeutic parenting (looked-after children are those taken into care due to neglect or abuse). This is based on an approach developed by the American psychologist Dan Hughes, which he calls PACE (Hughes, 2016). Playfulness, acceptance, curiosity and empathy are the foundations of an approach to parenting these traumatized children, alongside love. The deeply knowledgeable yoga teacher Jacquelyn Cooper was so enamoured by the concept of PACE that she made it the main theme of a yoga retreat for her students. However, everyone could benefit from improved interactions if they followed these principles. Indeed, we encourage our Yoga4Health teachers to display these qualities. We ask them not to be too serious and to occasionally be playful. We ask them to accept the patients as they are. We ask them to show curiosity about actions, reactions and interactions in class, rather than rushing to judgement. And we ask them to show empathy as people strive and, at times, struggle to develop the self-care skills they need.

In the group discussions at the end of each class, the technique of mirroring (verbally reflecting back to patients what they have expressed) supports an environment in which everyone feels heard. This is also an excellent skill to take out into life. When someone talks to you and you reflect back what they have said by summarizing their point of view, it can be remarkably affirming. They feel listened to. It is very different to waiting for a pause so that you can say what you think or reacting to what has been expressed by offering advice and trying to "fix" their problem.

When mirroring someone, we become better listeners and dearer friends. By really listening to what people are saying to us, we meet them and ourselves at a deeper level of connection. We become more observant and watchful about what is being said and our own reactions. This is likely to lead us to behaving in a more intelligent and compassionate way.

DIET

Official statistics show that 63% of the UK's population is overweight or obese, leading the government to publish a National Obesity Strategy in July 2020 (Department of Health and Social Care, 2021). *Tackling Obesity: Empowering Adults and Children to Live Healthier Lives* states: "Covid-19 has given us a wake-up call. We need to use this moment to kick start our health, get active and eat better."

The measures being implemented by the UK government include: providing tools and resources to help people lose weight; increasing NHS weight-management services; better labelling of foods; restricting volume promotions (like buy-one-get-one-free) on foods that are high in fat, sugar or salt; and banning the advertising of these products before the 9.00pm watershed.

The National Obesity Strategy recognizes that not enough has been done to tackle some of the underlying causes of preventable diseases linked to obesity, like cardiovascular disease and Type 2 diabetes. This view was echoed by the *Lancet*'s Editor, Dr Richard Horton, who wrote in October 2020 that for three decades governments around the world had failed to tackle the rise of preventable diseases and this had fuelled complications associated with the coronavirus pandemic and stalled life expectancy (Walker, 2020).

There is widespread evidence that a diet rich in fruits and vegetables, along with regular exercise and not smoking, all have a major impact on health. These measures lower the risks of developing lifestyle-related diseases like cardiovascular disease and Type 2 diabetes.

Food is a big issue for many people to deal with. On the one hand, it is simply mathematics. If you consume more calories in a day than you burn off, you will put on weight. You may have a genetic disposition to gain weight, but the same maths applies to all.

However, many of us seek emotional comfort in food – snacking on biscuits, crisps and other processed products between meals or in the evening. If we are feeling unhappy or unloved and without close family or a strong social network, we may experience an emptiness inside that we literally seek to fill with food.

Coming up with the next big thing in dieting has been a fast route to a bestselling book and getting rich quickly. However, how many of these diets have had a lasting effect? The experience of many people is that they follow the diet and lose weight but then relapse into old habits and put the weight back on.

In the journal *Nutrition*, in January 2020, Dr Rachel Freire undertook a systematic review of a range of diets aimed at weight loss and tackling obesity. She found that high-protein, low-carbohydrate diets and intermittent fasting were the most effective short-term ways to "jumpstart" weight loss (Freire, 2020). However, all diets were found to work if adhered to. Dr Freire concluded that it was "fundamental to adopt a diet that creates a negative energy balance [taking in fewer calories than you burn] and focuses on good food quality to promote health".

Adherence to a diet is also dependent on the ability of an individual to overcome the brain's "food reward" system. In an article by the University of Liverpool's Charlotte Hardman, an expert in the psychology of appetite, and Carl Roberts, a research fellow, they set out why the brain favours foods that are rich in energy and therefore calories (Hardman and Roberts, 2021). Junk food, like chocolate, ice cream, chips and cookies, are high in fat and sugar but also delicious. Our brains are wired to desire them, as such food sources were not readily available in the past, so high-calorie foods were very important. Hardman and Roberts say that:

> ...the nucleus accumbens (an area of the brain that controls motivation and reward) contains overlapping opioid and cannabinoid receptor sites that, when stimulated, produce powerful effects on desire, craving and food enjoyment.

The researchers continue that these systems of craving food appear to be more active in some people than others. Brain imaging studies have shown greater activity in the brain-reward regions of those who love chocolate than in those who are not chocoholics. These variations between individuals are yet to be explained, but they say it is likely to be a combination of genetic and learned factors.

The teachings of yoga suggest that an effective way of losing weight would be to tackle the source of overeating – the arising of the desire to overeat in the first place – while acknowledging that this process may be more challenging for some than others. This means refining the mind and being able to exercise judgement and wisdom in our responses to arising desires; this again is all about reflective practice and the gains that arise from it over time.

On the ten-week Yoga4Health programme we do not recommend a particular diet. Instead, lifestyle change arises naturally out of the cultivation of reflection and breath-and-body connection. Patients begin to feel more aware of their body and the sensations within it – when they are hungry, and when they are not. Patients begin to feel stronger, more flexible and healthier, and this leads them to make dietary choices to support that feeling. This probably explains why we had an unexpected 14 cm average reduction in waist measurement among the 279 NHS patients who participated in the programme in West London.

There's no point in going to yoga and then going and having spaghetti bolognese and three cakes and so it made you more aware of your body and what you were eating and how you were living. I genuinely believe that. (Cartwright *et al.*, 2019, p.29, patient focus group)

Yoga4Health patients also changed their diet:

Service users talked about how they became more aware of their eating habits and were able to change to healthier habits by reducing junk food and increasing fruit and vegetable consumption. Since practising yoga was seen as beneficial for health, unhealthy eating was seen to undermine practice. As a result, some participants described losing weight or reducing body fat content. Although less frequently reported than other benefits, this is supported by significant reductions in waist circumference. (Cartwright *et al.*, 2019, section 3.3.2)

The food we eat is shaped by our culture, family traditions, lifestyle (ready meals for those too busy to cook) and personal preferences. On the programme, patients undergo a guided journey of transformation. In terms of food, they are supported to find a pathway that works for them.

Becoming fully vegetarian or vegan is not for everyone. However, the health benefits of a mainly plant-based diet are compelling, and initiatives like Veganuary (eating vegan food for the whole of January) have grown in popularity. It is more likely that patients will improve their diets if they naturally feel the desire to make changes and then are supported by high-quality information about the most effective dietary changes that can be made.

For this reason, we do provide patients with information from Dean and Anne Ornish's *UnDo It!* book. There are seven evidence-based principles of healthy eating:

- Consume mostly plants: vegetables, fruits, whole grains, legumes, soy products, and small amounts of nuts and seeds in forms as close as possible to their natural, unprocessed state.

- What you include in your diet is as important as what you exclude. There are many thousands of protective factors in plant-based foods that have anti-cancer, anti-heart disease, and anti-aging properties as well as being very low in disease-pro-moting substances.

- Minimise or, even better, eliminate animal protein and replace it with plant-based protein.

- Avoid sugar, white flour, white rice, and other "bad carbs".

- Consume 3 grams per day of "good fats" (omega-3 fatty acids).

- Reduce intake of total fat, and especially "bad fats" such as trans fats, saturated fats, and partially hydrogenated fats.

- Organic is optional – foods taste much better, and they are much lower in pesticide residues, which can disrupt your hormones. (Ornish, 2019, p.62)

Dr Dixon is of the opinion that diet is the most important factor in promoting health. The college regularly runs Food As Medicine events on the health benefits of a diet rich in fruits and vegetables. Further information can be obtained from the College of Medicine and Integrated Health's website.

YOGA AS INTELLIGENT EXERCISE

Yoga is a highly intelligent form of physical exercise that methodically mobilizes all joints, stretches skeletal muscles and improves respiration, physical resilience, body systems and immune function.

However, most forms of exercise are beneficial, and many social-prescribing and community projects involve raising levels of physical activity. Local authority teams all over the UK are paid to provide support for, or directly organize, physical activity programmes in their area as part of their duty to promote public health.

In recent years, bodies like Sport England have focused more of their resources on grass-roots participation, as well as elite sport. This has seen inclusive activities like walking football and walking netball being offered to make the sedentary active again.

For those with a passion for sport, yoga has always been an excellent counterbalance to repetitive movements. For those seeking elevated heart rate for cardiovascular health, activities other than yoga can be complementary. Swimming is an effective way of building fitness while avoiding compression on joints. However, most active sports are preferable to inactivity which is so damaging to human health.

WELLBEING AND NATURE

In Week 10 of the Yoga4Health programme, we use the theme of connection to explore how patients link to themselves, their loved ones, their community and the planet. There is a growing body of evidence showing the mental and physical benefits of spending time in the natural world. A Danish study in 2019 found that children who grew up surrounded by green space were 55% less likely to develop a mental health disorder later in life (Engemann *et al.*, 2019). A systematic review of research into this area in the *Journal of Paediatric Nursing* in 2017 concluded that "access to green space was associated with improved mental well-being, overall health and cognitive development of children" (McCormick, 2017, p.3).

These findings are backed up by other studies covering adults and children. Barton and Pretty (2010) found that access to nature enhanced mood and self-esteem; Wells and Evans (2003) said that it acted as a buffer for daily stress; Bratman *et al.* (2019) found that preserving and enhancing opportunities for engagement with nature supports improved mental health.

For those in an urban environment, this may pose a challenge, although green spaces and parks abound in some cities. Moscow tops the list of cities with the most green space (54%), followed by Singapore City, Sydney and Vienna (WorldAtlas, 2021). In the UK, an aerial view of London reveals that it is dotted with much more green space than might be imagined.

Tony Juniper, in his book *What Has Nature Ever Done for Us?*, sets out the many ways in which "natural capital" underpins our way of life (Juniper, 2013). Degrade the environment and we are cutting the ground from beneath our feet, losing species and biodiversity at a rate that threatens ecosystem collapse, resulting in unprecedented economic costs.

An important part of the story of becoming more aware, grounded and rooted in yoga is reconnecting with nature and taking pleasure in the simple – and free – things that life has to offer. There are few things more nourishing than being in an unspoilt forest or among majestic mountains and oceans. And few activities more relaxing than walking or sitting by a beautiful river. Being in nature forces us to slow down and simply become absorbed and connected to what is around us. To admire the trees, birds and wildlife and feel that ancient connection to the natural world rekindled.

Stress costs the NHS and healthcare systems around the world billions of pounds every year. Schemes promoting access to nature could be a cost-effective way of reducing stress and its symptoms and boosting quality of life. Juniper urges us to make use of what he calls "this Natural Health Service" (Juniper, 2013, p.245).

Yoga practice creates connections between the individual and their body and breath, but also with others, with community and ultimately with the world. Yoga practitioners who make lifestyle changes often gravitate towards an appreciation of the natural world and a desire to support groups working in conservation. Yoga means union and oneness. The wider expression of this can be to feel our connection to everyone and everything on our Earth and in our Universe.

FINAL THOUGHTS

Our aspiration for Yoga4Health was to create a programme that would give patients a yoga toolkit. Not a set of techniques that can only be practised on a yoga mat or in a chair, but a set of practical tools for life. Some may be drawn to the postures, others the breathing, relaxation or meditation. Whatever a person is drawn to, we hope they integrate the skills that speak to them in their daily lives. This might mean practising mindful breathing in the supermarket queue or teaching a stressed-out friend the long exhale or Coherent Breathing, or making yoga an indelible part of every morning. Through this, we hope all who join our programme slowly move to a place of greater and greater wellbeing through their own volition and a deeper connection with themselves and others.

REFERENCES

Barton, J. and Pretty, J. (2010). 'What is the best dose of nature and green exercise for improving mental health? A multi-study analysis.' *Environmental Science & Technology 44*, 10, 3947–3955.

Bratman, G. N., Anderson, C. B., Berman, M. G., Cochran, B., *et al.* (2019). 'Nature and mental health: An ecosystem service perspective.' *Science Advances 5*, 7.

Cartwright, T., Richards, R., Edwards, A. and Cheshire, A. (2019). *Yoga4Health on Social Prescription: A Mixed Methods Evaluation.* London: University of Westminster.

Department of Health and Social Care (2021). *Tackling Obesity: Empowering Adults and Children to Live Healthier Lives.* Accessed on 16/9/2021 at: www. gov.uk/government/publications/tackling-obesity-government-strategy/ tackling-obesity-empowering-adults-and-children-to-live-healthier-lives.

Engemann, K., Pedersen, C. B., Arge, L., Tsirogiannis, C., Mortensen, P. B. and Svenning, J. C. (2019). 'Residential green space in childhood is associated with lower risk of psychiatric disorders from adolescence into adulthood.' *Proceedings of the National Academy of Sciences of the United States of America 116*, 11, 5188–5193.

Freire, D. R. (2020). 'Scientific evidence of diets for weight loss.' *Nutrition*, 110549.

Hardman, C. and Roberts, C. H. (2021). *Here's Why We Crave Food Even When We're Not Hungry.* Accessed on 16/9/2021 at: https://theconversation.com/ heres-why-we-crave-food-even-when-were-not-hungry-144238.

Hawley, J. (2012). *The Bhagavad Gita: A Walkthrough for Westerners.* Novato, CA: New World Library.

Hughes, D. (2016). *Parenting a Child Who Has Experienced Trauma.* London: Coram.

Juniper, T. (2013). *What Has Nature Ever Done for Us?* London: Profile Books.

McCormick, R. (2017). 'Does access to green space impact the mental well-being of children? A systematic review.' *Journal of Paediatric Nursing 37*, 3–7.

Olivelle, P. (2008). *Upanishads.* Oxford: Oxford University Press.

Ornish, D. A. (2019). *UnDo It!* New York: Ballantine Books, Random House.

Stiles, M. (2001). *Yoga Sutras of Patanjali.* Boston, MA: Red Wheel.

Walker, T. (2020). *Preventable Lifestyle Diseases are Driving COVID-19 and We Need a Radical Change of Direction to Deal With It, says The Lancet.* Accessed on 15/10/2021 at: www.leisureopportunities.co.uk/news/COVID-19-pandemic-The-Lancet-Richard-Horton/346450.

Wells, N. M. and Evans, G. W. (2003). 'Nearby nature: A buffer of life stress among rural children.' *Environment and Behaviour 35*, 3, 311–330.

WorldAtlas (2021). *Cities With the Most Green Space.* Accessed on 15/10/2021 at: www. worldatlas.com/articles/cities-with-the-most-greenspace.html#:~:text=Cities%20 With%20The%20Most%20Green%20Space%201%20Moscow.,Australia.%20...%20 4%20Vienna.%20...%205%20Shenzhen.%20.

Epilogue

Readers outside the UK may be thinking, "It's fine for them, but what about us?" It is true that social prescribing has developed further and faster in the UK than anywhere else in the world. However, that is all beginning to change.

The UK's Social Prescribing Network's annual event has become the International Social Prescribing Network conference, with examples and awards for innovative and effective projects in many countries. These include the United States, Canada, Australia, New Zealand, Singapore, Republic of Ireland, Portugal and the Western Pacific Region. All have presented their work at the conference.

In the US, the Veterans Association has shown how a range of complementary therapies offered at scale in thousands of healthcare settings can have a dramatic impact on health and wellness. Interventions like yoga and meditation have been championed by the Whole Health Institute and the Chopra Research Library. Countless organizations and individual yoga teachers are already offering yoga as social prescribing, even if it currently goes by another name.

This is no surprise. Complementary therapies and mind-body practices have been around for centuries. What is new is the solidifying evidence base, the vocabulary to engage with healthcare professionals in a language they understand, and the realization that the sustainability of healthcare systems everywhere will increasingly depend on strategies that include patient activation and promoting self-care. Social prescribing offers an accessible, simple and transferable model to enable policy makers and healthcare leaders to tackle the big problems they face: non-communicable diseases, including greater physical activity and tackling the mental health crisis by reducing stress and anxiety and improving mood.

Yoga provides an astoundingly effective set of tools through posture, breathwork, mindfulness and meditation to address these problems of the age. Armed with these beautiful and powerful practices, yoga teachers working in healthcare have the potential to make deep inroads into improving people's physical and mental health for the benefit of all. One of the most appropriate vehicles for them to use to make this progress is social prescribing.

Our call to action for those yoga teachers living in areas of the world where social prescribing is in its infancy is to use this book to sow the seeds, make the connections and build the network from the ground up. The data is compelling, the need is great and we believe that you will find fertile ground wherever you are.

We here at the Yoga in Healthcare Alliance are ready to support you in every way that we can (visit www.yogainhealthcarealliance.com or email contactyoga4health@gmail.com).

Resources

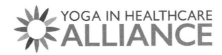

If you are an experienced yoga teacher or health professional interested in training to deliver the Yoga4Health protocol please visit www.yoga inhealthcarealliance.com or email contactyoga4health@gmail.com.

College of Medicine and Integrated Health
www.collegeofmedicine.org.uk

Academic Consortium for Integrative Medicine & Health
www.imconsortium.org

The Minded Institute
www.themindedinstitute.com

University of Westminster
www.westminster.ac.uk

Mediyoga
www.mediyoga.se

Ayush
www.ayush.gov.in

NHS
www.nhs.uk

Public Health England
www.gov.uk/government/organisations/public-health-england

Centers for Disease Control and Prevention – US
www.cdc.gov

World Health Organization
www.who.int

PubMed – Research Papers
www.pubmed.ncbi.nlm.nih.gov

The British Wheel of Yoga
www.bwy.org.uk

Yoga Scotland
www.yogascotland.org.uk

Yoga Alliance
www.yogaalliance.org

British Council for Yoga Therapy
www.bcyt.org

International Association of Yoga Therapists
www.iayt.org

Breath-Body-Mind
www.breath-body-mind.com

Harvard Medical School
www.hms.harvard.edu

Whole Health Institute
www.wholehealth.org

Coherent Breathing
https://coherentbreathing.com

Buteyko Clinic International
www.buteykoclinic.com

FURTHER READING

Alexander, G. K., Innes, K. E., Selfe, T. K. and Brown, C. J. (2013). 'More than I expected: Perceived benefits of yoga practice among older adults at risk of cardiovascular disease.' *Complementary Therapies in Medicine 21*, 14–28.

American Heart Association (2017). 'Unhealthy diets linked to more than 400,000 cardiovascular deaths.' *American Heart Association Meeting Report Presentation 15*. Accessed on 9/9/2021 at: www.eurekalert.org/pub_releases/2017-03/aha-udl030117.php.

Benson, H. (2007). *The Relaxation Response.* London: William Morrow & Co.

Chong, C. S., Tsunaka, M. and Chan, E. P. (2011). 'Effects of yoga on stress management in healthy adults: A systematic review.' *Alternative Therapies in Health and Medicine 17*, 32.

Cramer, H., Lauche, R., Haller, H., Steckhan, N., Michalsen, A. and Dobos, G. (2014). 'Effects of yoga on cardiovascular disease risk factors: A systematic review and meta-analysis.' *International Journal of Cardiology 173*, 170–183.

Cramer, H., Lauche, R., Langhorst, J. and Dobos, G. (2013). 'Yoga for depression: A systematic review and meta-analysis.' *Depression and Anxiety 30*, 1068–1083.

Gabriel, M. G., Curtiss, J., Hofmann, S. G. and Khalsa, S. (2018). 'Kundalini yoga for generalized anxiety disorder: An exploration of treatment efficacy and possible mechanisms.' *International Journal of Yoga Therapy 28*, 1, 97–105.

Haider, T., Sharma, M. and Branscum, P. (2017). 'Yoga as an alternative and complimentary therapy for cardiovascular disease.' *Journal of Evidence-Based Complementary and Alternative Medicine 22*, 2, 310–316.

Hartley, L., Dyakova, M., Holmes, J., Clarke, A., *et al.* (2014). 'Yoga for the primary prevention of cardiovascular disease.' *The Cochrane Database of Systematic Reviews 5*, CD010072.

International Diabetes Federation (2020). *Diabetes Facts and Figures.* Accessed on 9/9/2021 at: www.idf.org/aboutdiabetes/what-is-diabetes/facts-figures.html.

Kim, H.-S. K. (2017). 'Effects of relaxation therapy on anxiety disorders: A systematic review and meta-analysis.' *Archives of Psychiatric Nursing*, 278–284.

Kinser, P. A., Bourguignon, C., Taylor, A. G. and Steeves, R. (2013). 'A feeling of connectedness: Perspectives on a gentle yoga intervention for women with major depression.' *Issues in Mental Health Nursing 34*, 402–411.

Kishida, M., Mana, S. K., Larkey, L. K. and Elavsky, S. (2018). 'Yoga resets my inner peace barometer: A qualitative study illuminating the pathways of how yoga impacts one's relationship to oneself and to others.' *Complementary Therapies in Medicine 40*, 215–221.

Lindahl, E., Tilton, K., Eickholt, N. and Ferguson-Stegall, L. (2016). 'Yoga reduces perceived stress and exhaustion levels in healthy elderly individuals.' *Complementary Therapies in Clinical Practice 24*, 50–56.

Pascoe, M. C. and Bauer, I. E. (2015). 'A systematic review of randomised control trials on the effects of yoga on stress measures and mood.' *Journal of Psychiatric Research 68*, 270–282.

Pascoe, M. C., Thompson, D. R. and Ski, C. F. (2017). 'Yoga, mindfulness-based stress reduction and stress-related physiological measures: A meta-analysis.' *Psychoneuroendocrinology 86*, 152–168.

Porges, S. (2011). *The Polyvagal Theory: Neurophysiological Foundations of Emotion, Attachment, Communication and Self-Regulation.* New York: Norton.

Ross, A., Bevans, M., Friedmann, E., Williams, L. and Thomas, S. (2014). 'I am a nice person when I do yoga!!!' *Journal of Holistic Nursing 32*, 67–77.

Simon, N. M., Hofmann, S. G., Rosenfield, D., Hoeppner, S. S., *et al.* (2021). 'Efficacy of yoga vs cognitive behavioral therapy vs stress education for the treatment of generalized anxiety disorder: A randomized clinical trial.' *JAMA Psychiatry 78*, 1, 13–20.
Singleton, J. M. (2017). *Roots of Yoga.* London: Penguin.
Streeter, C. C., Gerbarg, P. L., Saper, R. B., Ciraulo, D. A. and Brown, R. P. (2012). 'Effects of yoga on the autonomic nervous system, gamma-aminobutyric-acid, and allostasis in epilepsy, depression, and post-traumatic stress disorder.' *Medical Hypotheses 78*, 5, 571–579.
Thind, H., Lantini, R., Balletto, B. L., Donahue, M. L., *et al.* (2017). 'The effects of yoga among adults with type 2 diabetes: A systematic review and meta-analysis.' *Preventive Medicine 105*, 116–126.

About the Authors

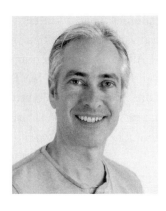

Paul Fox has been a British Wheel of Yoga (BWY) teacher since 1999 and has trained over 200 people to become BWY yoga teachers. Paul is passionate about social prescribing and the opportunity to bring yoga to individuals and communities not currently served. In all his teaching he offers both chair and mat instructions. He also holds yoga teaching qualifications in Ashtanga Vinyasa Yoga and is a Yoga Sports Science Yoga Sports Coach. Paul has well over 1000 hours of continuing professional development and holds the Post-Graduate Certificate in Education (PGCE). While Chair of BWY, he championed diversity, inclusion and standards. He also led the Ofqual-regulated awarding organization British Wheel of Yoga Qualifications (BWYQ). Since 2016, Paul has played a leading role with Heather Mason in developing the work of the Yoga in Healthcare Alliance, including training and supporting over 225 Yoga4Health teachers. He published the yoga novel *Yoga Quest* in 2016 and is working on a book with Emma Conally-Barklem to present Ashtanga Vinyasa Yoga in a completely accessible form.

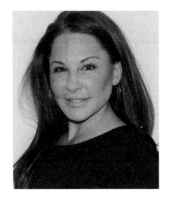

Heather Mason is the founder of The Minded Institute, a leading yoga therapy training school in the UK, and the founding director of the Yoga in Healthcare Alliance. Committed to bringing yoga into health systems, she has also taught in medical schools, educating future doctors in integrating yoga into treatment, created the first mind-body medicine course on the US's first Master of Science Degree in Yoga Therapy at the Maryland University of Integrated Health, developed various programmes for yoga's integration into healthcare and continues to lecture at various universities on this topic. Heather is the secretariate for the All-Party Parliamentary Group on Yoga in Society in the UK. She is an RYT-500 and C-IAYT; holds MAs in Psychotherapy and Buddhist Studies and an MS in Medical Physiology; and has done extensive study in neuroscience. She is also the Co-Editor of the core text for yoga in mental healthcare: *Yoga for Mental Health*.

Index